Foreword

D0523665

The need for First Aid training is greater than ever. ~ ~p~~
are growing throughout the world, and the increased use of
mechanical and electrical appliances in everyday use, at
home, at work and at play, places more and more people at
risk of injury.

There is thus an evergrowing demand for First Aid training
for personal use, quite apart from the demand for Certificated
First Aiders as part of industrial and commercial establish-
ments.

The Authorised Joint First Aid Manual of the three
Voluntary Aid Societies sets out to provide the material for
instructional courses to achieve proficiency certificates. It is
an instructional Manual and work of reference designed to
meet the needs of those with a serious interest in First Aid
training, who require an acknowledged qualification.

Great care has been taken in the preparation of the 3rd
edition, to obtain the views of the widest spread of First
Aid users, and this has involved consultation with leading
authorities in all fields, both at home and abroad, so as to
make the work as universally acceptable as is possible. For
all this help the Voluntary Aid Societies are much indebted.
They recognise that it is impossible to produce a work in
any field which will secure the immediate and unreserved
approval of all readers, and First Aid is no exception. But at
the same time, it is hoped that it will be recognised that great
care has been taken to evaluate the material considered by
the Revision Committee, and that as comprehensive a view
as is consistent with clear teaching has been applied.

The Committee has accepted the general view that the
material for the Standard Adult First Aid Certificate should be
presented separately bound within its own covers, and is
confident that the Medical Lecturers and Lay Instructors, on
whom so much of the three Societies' work depends, will
find themselves equipped with a simple, clear and
authoritative text.

The St. John Ambulance Association and Brigade

St. Andrew's Ambulance Association

The British Red Cross Society

Contents

Note on examination requirements

This Manual provides the material for the standard First Aid Course, leading to the award of the First Aid Certificate issued by each of the Voluntary Aid Societies, which is recognized for certain statutory purposes. The Appendices do not form part of the course, and in the examination, no questions will be based on this material. The three Societies promulgate separately their own conditions and requirements leading to the award of Higher Certificates and Certificates of Advanced Knowledge, but in all cases possession of the statutory First Aid Certificate is an essential pre-requisite to the gaining of higher qualifications.

Changing social conditions, involving greater competition for leisure time have made inroads on the traditional pattern of First Aid training carried out in weekly 2-hour or $2\frac{1}{2}$-hour sessions. There is a trend towards the week-end school type of instruction; and this is increasing. For Industrial purposes there is a demand for Intensive instruction, where the course is delivered over four full days. The 6-session and 8-session presentations of the syllabus which follow, therefore, are recommended as a guide only, and each Society approves suitable alternative arrangements as requisite.

SYLLABUS

Six-Session Presentation
(2$\frac{1}{2}$-hour sessions)

SESSION 1

THEORETICAL (Chapters 1, 2, 3, 4)
Principles and practice of First Aid
Action at an emergency
Structure and functions of the body*
Dressings and bandages
  *Not required for examination purposes.

PRACTICAL (Chapter 4, Pages 50-67)
Bandages and their application
  Triangular
  Prepared Roller
  Tubular gauze
  Elasticised net
  Slings

SESSION 2

THEORETICAL (Chapters 5, 6, 7)
Asphyxia and emergency resuscitation
Wounds, bleeding and circulatory failure
Shock

PRACTICAL (Chapters 5, 6)
Resuscitation:—
  Mouth to mouth method
  Holger Nielsen method
  External heart Compression
  Recovery position
(Chapter 6, Pages 48-67)
Application of dressings and bandages –
  continued
(Chapter 6, Pages 90-101)
Pressure points
Control of bleeding

SESSION 3

THEORETICAL (Chapters 8, 9)
Injuries to bones
Injuries to muscles, ligaments and joints

PRACTICAL (Chapter 8, Pages 121-126)
Management of fractures (upper limbs)
(Chapter 9, Pages 135-138)
Injuries to muscles, ligaments, joints
Dislocations

SESSION 4

THEORETICAL (Chapters 10, 11)
The nervous system and unconsciousness
Burns and scalds

PRACTICAL (Chapter 8, Pages 127-134)
Management of fractures (lower limbs)
(Pages 115-120)
Management of fractured spine

SESSION 5

THEORETICAL (Chapters 12, 13)
Poisoning
Miscellaneous conditions

PRACTICAL (Chapter 15, Pages 178-200)
Handling and transport of injured persons
(Chapter 8, Pages 115-120)
Fractured Spine (revision)
(Pages 121-134)
Fractures, upper and lower limbs (revision)

SESSION 6

THEORETICAL (Chapters 14, 15)
Procedure at road accidents
Handling and transport of injured persons

SESSION 6 – continued

PRACTICAL REVISION PERIOD
(Chapter 4, Pages 50-67)
Bandages and their application
(Chapter 6, Pages 48-67)
Application of dressings and bandages

Pressure points and control of bleeding
(Chapters 5, 6, Pages 68-80, Page 17 Fig 2)
Resuscitation all methods
External heart compression
Recovery position

Eight-Session Presentation
(2 hour sessions)

SESSION 1
THEORETICAL *(Chapters 1 and 2)*
Principles and practice of First Aid
Responsibility of a First Aider – Assessment
and initial action; diagnosis
Principles of treatment
Priorities – dangers and urgent needs; other
needs
Disposal and report
Structure and functions of the body
(Chapter 3)
General principles
Practical
Examination of a casualty
Turning and positioning of unconscious
casualty in 'recovery position'

SESSION 2
The respiratory system and asphyxia
(Chapters 3 and 5)
The lungs, air passages and diaphragm
The mechanism of breathing
Asphyxia and its causes
Emergency Resuscitation

SESSION 3
Shock *(Chapter 7)*
The circulatory system and bleeding
(Chapters 3 and 6)
Blood and the circulation;
Wounds and Bleeding; Control of bleeding
Bleeding from special areas
(Chapter 4)
Application of dressing and bandages

SESSION 4
**The circulatory system and bleeding
(continued)** *(Chapters 4 and 6)*
Bleeding from special areas *(continued)*
Circulatory failure
Dressings and bandages *(continued)*
including improvisation
Simple methods of carrying
(Chapter 15)

SESSION 5
**The nervous system and
unconsciousness**
(Chapters 10 and 7)
The nervous system
Unconsciousness
Fainting
Poisoning
(Chapter 12)

SESSION 6
Burns and scalds
(Chapter 11)
Burns and scalds
Corrosive injuries
Electrical burns
Injuries to bones
(Chapter 8)
Fractures – causes, types, signs and
symptoms; general rules for treatment
Transport – stretcher loading and carrying
(Chapter 15)

SESSION 7
**Injuries to bones (continued), muscles,
ligaments, joints**
(Chapters 8 and 9)
Special fractures
Strains, sprains and dislocations;
displaced cartilage of knee
Transport *(continued)* including
improvisation

SESSION 8
Miscellaneous conditions
(Chapters 13 and 14)
Miscellaneous conditions
Procedure at road accidents
A practical incident
NOTE: Bandages, slings and transport should
be introduced as appropriate and practised
throughout the course.

CHAPTER ONE

Principles and practice of First Aid

First Aid is the skilled application of accepted principles of treatment on the occurrence of an accident or in the case of sudden illness, using facilities or materials available at the time.

It is the approved method of treating a casualty until he is placed, if necessary, in the care of a doctor or removed to hospital.

Because of the increasing number and serious nature of accidents of all kinds, the responsibility of the First Aider has become greater.

First Aid is treatment given to a casualty –
– to sustain life.
– to prevent his condition from becoming worse.
– to promote his recovery.

Responsibility of a First Aider in the management of a casualty

To **assess** the situation;

To arrive at a **diagnosis** for each casualty;

To give immediate and adequate **treatment,** bearing in mind that a casualty may have more than one injury and that some casualties will require more urgent attention than others;

To arrange without delay for the **disposal** of a casualty according to the seriousness of his condition.

Assessment and initial action

Be calm, take charge.
Give confidence to the conscious casualty.
Talk to him, listen to him and reassure him.

Check –
– safety of casualties and of yourself;
– the breathing, for bleeding and whether conscious.

7

Get others to help.
Tell them what they should do.
If necessary, send for ambulance, police, fire service, or other help.

Diagnosis

The *history* of the incident must be taken into consideration, and an examination made to determine the *signs* and *symptoms*, and *level of consciousness*.

History
The story of how the accident happened or the illness began obtained from –
The casualty: 'I slipped and fell down'.
A Witness: 'I saw the old.man fall and his head strike the wall'.

Signs
Variations from normal, ascertained by the First Aider – Pallor; blueness (*cyanosis*) of face, lips, inner sides of eyelids, or of nail beds of fingers and toes.
There may be evidence of poisoning.

Symptoms
Sensations described by the casualty –
'I feel pain'.
'I am cold'.
'My arm is numb'.

Level of consciousness

Any change of level is important.
Full consciousness
Able to speak and answer questions normally.

Drowsiness
Easily roused, but lapses into unconsciousness.

Stupor
Can be roused with difficulty. The casualty is aware of painful stimuli, e.g. pin prick, but not of other external events, e.g. being spoken to.

Coma
Cannot be roused by any stimuli.

Action

If the cause of the condition is still active, remove it –
– a log of wood on the casualty's leg,
– contaminated clothing

8

or, remove the casualty from the cause — from traffic, fire, water, poisonous fumes etc.

Treatment

Give the treatment you consider essential.
Sustain life.
Emergency resuscitation*.
Control bleeding and shock.

Prevent the condition from becoming worse.
Cover wounds.
Immobilise fractures, large wounds and any injured part.
Place the casualty in a correct and comfortable position.

Promote recovery.
Reassure.
Give any other treatment needed.
Relieve pain.
Handle gently and carefully at all times.
Move as little as possible.
Protect from cold.

Disposal

The First Aider will ensure that the casualty is conveyed without delay to his home, a suitable shelter or an appropriate hospital. In serious cases it may be necessary to summon a doctor.
A brief written report should accompany the casualty.
A tactful message should also be sent, if necessary, to the casualty's home stating what has happened and where he has been taken, unless this has been done by the police or other authority.

Summary of essentials of First Aid

Act quickly, quietly and methodically, giving priority to the most urgent conditions.
Ensure that there is no further danger to the casualty or to yourself.
If breathing has stopped or is failing, clear the airway and, if necessary, start emergency resuscitation.

* *If in doubt as to whether or not the casualty is dead, give treatment —*
— until medical aid is available, or
— until stiffening of the muscles (rigor mortis) after death commences, or
— to the limits of your own physical capacity.

Control bleeding.

Determine the level of consciousness.

Consider the possibility of poisoning.

Give reassurance as necessary to the casualty and to those around and so help to lessen anxiety.

Guard against shock.

Position the casualty correctly.

Before moving the casualty, immobilise fractures and large wounds.

Arrange without delay for the careful conveyance of the casualty, if necessary, to the care of his doctor or to a hospital.

Watch and record any changes in the condition of the casualty.

Do not attempt too much;

Do not allow people to crowd round: this hinders first aid and may cause the casualty anxiety or embarrassment;

Do not remove clothing unnecessarily;

Do not give anything by mouth to a casualty who is unconscious, who has a suspected internal injury, or who may shortly need an anaesthetic.

Definitions

Medical aid indicates treatment by a doctor.

First Aider: The term First Aider was devised to designate 'any person who has received a certificate from an authorised Association that he or she is qualified to render First Aid'. It was first used in this way in 1894 by the Voluntary First Aid Organisations.

Such certificates issued by St. John Ambulance, St. Andrew's Ambulance Association and British Red Cross Society are awarded to candidates who have attended a course of theoretical and practical work, and who have passed an examination conducted by a specially appointed doctor.

The certificate awarded has a limited validity of three years thus ensuring that First Aiders are —

— highly trained;

— regularly examined;

— kept up-to-date in knowledge and skill.

CHAPTER TWO

Action at an emergency

The First Aider must be prepared to take responsibility.
This includes –
– an appreciation of the situation;
– taking charge until someone more experienced is available;
– diagnosis;
– treatment and disposal.

Multiple casualties

Where there is more than one casualty, the First Aider must decide by rapid assessment, which one should receive priority of treatment.

Consideration must be given to –
– the immediate placing of any unconscious casualties in the **recovery position** (previously known as the coma

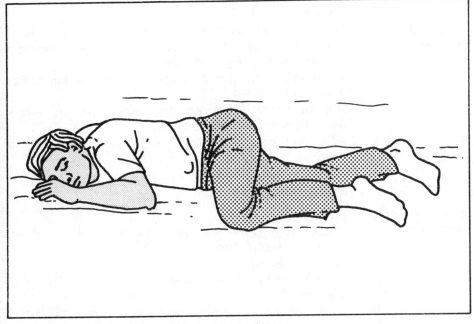

Figure 1: The recovery position

11

position and, earlier, as the three quarters prone position);
– temporary control of continuous severe bleeding with the assistance of the casualty, or by a bystander, if available;
– restoration of breathing, if necessary.

A First Aider working alone must quickly place all unconscious casualties in the recovery position before attending to any others.

Note: The noisiest casualty need not be the most severely injured!

Bystanders

Make use of any bystanders; keep them occupied—the more they are given to do, the less they will interfere. They should be used to telephone for the ambulance, police or any other service, to keep back any crowds which may gather, to assist with the control of traffic at a road accident, and, if necessary, to assist with the actual treatment of the casualty.

When sending bystanders to telephone, make sure that they understand the message to be sent; write it down if possible, but in any case ask them to repeat the message (before actually sending it).

Priorities

Danger to the casualty

The First Aider must first reduce to a minimum any danger to the casualty or to himself (take care to avoid becoming a second casualty), e.g. in the case of –
– *road accidents:* instruct someone to control the traffic; reference chapter 14
– *electrocution:* switch off the current; take necessary precautions against electric shock;
– *fire and collapsing buildings:* move the casualty to safety;
—*gas and poisonous fumes:* turn off at source, remove casualty to fresh air.

Urgent needs of the casualty

Breathing
Check that his airway is clear and that he is breathing; if not, commence artificial respiration.
Unconsciousness
Place him in the recovery position.
Bleeding
Check for serious bleeding and control it; raise the part if possible and if no fracture is suspected.

Other needs

When these urgent matters have received attention, time can be taken to obtain the history of the accident, to weigh up the situation, and to decide in which order action should be taken.

Establish the level of consciousness;

immobilise all serious fractures and large wounds before moving the casualty, unless there is immediate danger to life from the surroundings;

give appropriate treatment to the condition found.

Ambulance or medical aid

Immediately it is decided that an ambulance is required, send for it, stating —

— the exact place of the accident (if necessary with directions of how to get there);

— the number, and approximate age of the casualties;

— some indication of the type and seriousness of the accident, e.g. car crash, fall from building, the nature of the injury or injuries.

In all cases of suspected fracture of the spine, or heart attack, obtain medical aid, if readily available, or transport to hospital immediately. In country districts a doctor may be obtained more quickly than an ambulance.

Diagnosis

Use all your senses to obtain maximum information — look, speak, listen, feel and smell.

Conscious casualty

If the casualty is conscious —

— look and size up the problem as you approach;

— ask him if he has pain and where it is; examine that part first;

— ask him if he thinks there is anything else wrong;

— handle injured parts gently but firmly;

— make sure there are no other injuries present, which may be masked by pain, by checking for tenderness and bleeding;

— examine the casualty carefully in a regular and methodical manner by running your hands gently but firmly over all parts of the body. Start at the head and neck, then check the spine and trunk; the upper limbs, the lower limbs.

Always compare abnormal parts with the normal side.

13

The First Aider need only remove enough of the casualty's clothing to expose the injuries and treat them.

Then check —
– colour of skin, the nail beds and the inside of the eyelids;
– the nature of the breathing – listen to it: smell the breath;
– count the pulse – noting its strength and rhythm;
– the temperature of the body – whether hot or cold to the touch.

Unconscious casualty

If the casualty is unconscious —
– the task is much more difficult and a thorough detailed examination is necessary;
– note if breathing is present: if absent, immediately commence artificial respiration;
– examine over and under the casualty for dampness which might indicate bleeding. Stop any serious bleeding before proceeding further with the examination;
– bear in mind the possibility of internal bleeding;
– establish the cause of unconsciousness by examining the —
– *breathing* – rate and depth;
– *pulse* – rate and character;
– *face and skin* – colour, temperature and condition;
– *pupils* of the eyes;
– *head* for injury;
– *ears, eyes, nose and mouth* for blood and other signs;
– *whole body* for signs of injury.

Treatment

Carry out the appropriate treatment gently and quickly in a confident manner. *Reassurance* and *encouragement* of the casualty is most important – calmness and efficiency on the part of the First Aider will inspire greater confidence than mere words. *Common sense is essential on every occasion.*

Pay attention to the casualty's requests and any remarks he may make – remember the casualty may overhear remarks not intended for him.

When the appropriate treatment has been given, keep a careful watch on the casualty until he has been sent to hospital or is no longer the responsibility of the First Aider.

*Do **not*** pester the casualty by asking repeatedly how he is feeling. This is most annoying and a sign of nervousness on the part of the First Aider.

Disposal

After the First Aider has carried out his treatment, the casualty may be –
– sent to hospital by ambulance, or in appropriate cases, by car;
– handed over to the care of a doctor, a nurse or other responsible person;
– taken into a nearby house or shelter to await the arrival of ambulance or doctor;
– allowed to go home and told to seek medical advice, if necessary.

Note: Do not send anyone home unaccompanied who has been *unconscious,* if only for a short period, or is badly *shocked*.

Report on casualty

Hospital and medical authorities should be informed. If the ambulance does not carry a two-way communication system, use a label or written message to explain the circumstances of the accident or illness and the treatment given.

Be brief – use the least number of words which will convey your meaning clearly. *Do not* use abbreviations.

When sending a message by telephone ask the person receiving the message to repeat it to make sure that it has been fully understood.

Before disposing of the casualty take his name and address and also that of the nearest relative or friend and check that an appropriate message is being sent to them by the police or other authority.

Take care of any personal property of the casualty and hand this over to the police or ambulance personnel before leaving the site of the incident.

Removal of clothing

Remove only sufficient clothing to expose injuries and to treat them.
Such removal should be done with a minimum of disturbance to the casualty and to clothing.
Do not damage clothing unnecessarily.

In some instances it may be necessary to cut women's underclothing, if tight.

Method

Coat
Raise the casualty and slip the coat over his shoulders; then bend the arm on the sound side and remove from that side first. If necessary, slit up the seam on the injured side.

Shirt and vest
Remove as for the coat. If necessary, slit the shirt down the front.

Trousers
Pull down from the waist or raise trouser leg as required. If necesssary, slit up the seam.

Boot or shoe
Steady the ankle, undo or cut the laces and remove carefully.
If the casualty is wearing long boots, carefully slit up the seam with a sharp knife or razor blade.

Socks
If difficult to remove, insert two fingers between the sock and the leg, raise the edge of the sock and cut it between your fingers.

Turning a casualty

It may be necessary to turn a casualty when lying on his back into the **recovery position**. This can be done as follows:—

1. Kneel beside him and place both his arms close to his body.

2. Turn the casualty gently on to his side (this may conveniently be done by grasping the clothing at the hip).

3. Draw up the upper arm until it makes a right angle with the body and bend the elbow.

4. Draw up the upper leg until the thigh makes a right angle with the body and bend the knee.

5. Draw out the underneath arm gently backwards to extend slightly behind his back.

6. Bend the undermost knee slightly.

The effect of placing the limbs in this manner provides the necessary stability to keep the casualty comfortable in the

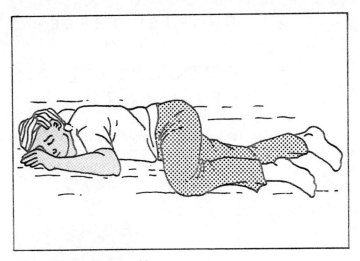

Figure 2: The recovery position

recovery position. With his head turned to one side the possibility of vomit causing drowning (asphyxia) is eliminated.

If the casualty is a heavy person, two hands may be necessary to grasp the clothing and in this instance the First Aider should kneel at the side of the casualty so that when he is turned his face will rest against the First Aider's knees. If bystanders are present make use of them to protect the casualty's face and assist in the turning.

CHAPTER THREE

Structure and functions of the body

In order to understand and apply the principles of First Aid

Figure 3: The skeleton

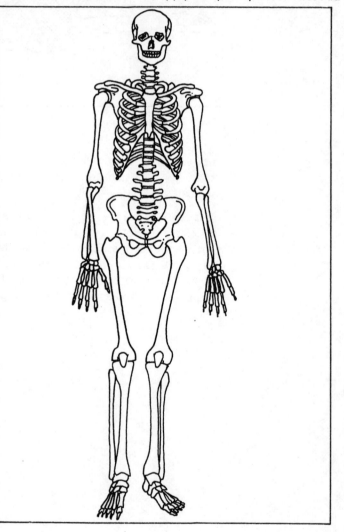

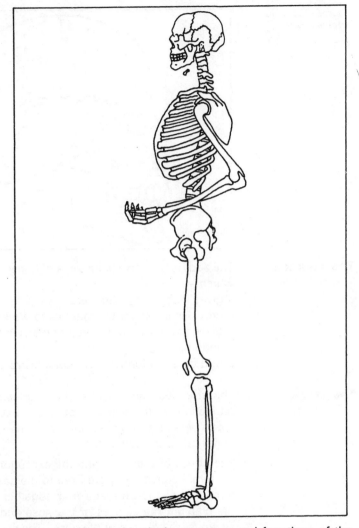

some knowledge of both the structure and functions of the body is necessary.

Structure of the body

The body consists of different kinds of materials called 'tissues' which consist of a multitude of tiny units called 'cells'.

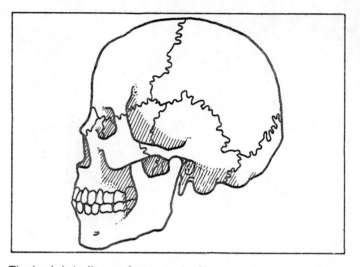

Figure 5: The skull, left side view

The skeleton

The body is built on a framework of bones called the **skeleton** which –
– gives it shape and firmness;
– provides levers for the muscles to work;
– gives protection to important organs in the skull, chest and abdomen.
Blood cells are formed from bone marrow.

The skull

The rounded part of the skull (*cranium*) forms a rigid protection for the brain. Through the base of the skull pass blood vessels and nerves, including the large mass of nerve fibres called the spinal cord.

The bones of the face, with the exception of the lower jaw, are firmly united. They are fixed to the base or bottom of the front part of the skull and form together with the bones of the cranium the cavities of the nose and eyes; contain the air sinuses and support the nose. The cavity of the mouth is between the upper and lower jaws, the palate being the bony roof of the mouth which separates it from the nose.

The upper jaw bone has sockets for the upper teeth.

The lower jaw bone consists of a horizontal portion, in which are sockets for the lower teeth, and two vertical portions terminating and hinging on to each side of the base of the skull in front of the ear. The junction of the horizontal and

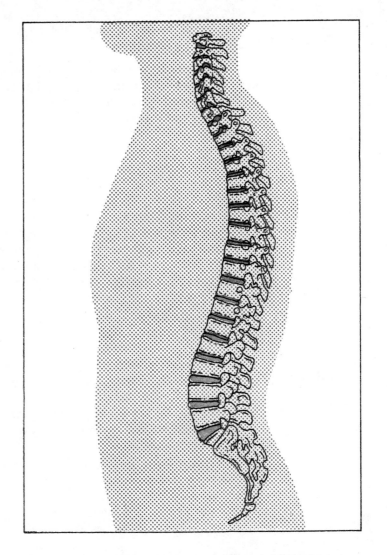

Figure 6: Vertebral column, with discs, left side view

each vertical portion is known as the angle of the jaw.

Spine or backbone

The spine (*vertebral column*) is formed of thirty-three bones called vertebrae.

The body of each vertebra consists of a bony mass, from the back of which two separate bony processes project and unite in the shape of an arch, so forming the spinal canal through which runs the spinal cord.

The tip of the arch of each vertebra can be felt by running a finger down the spine.

The vertebrae are grouped in regions in each of which they are known by numbers, counting downwards –
– in the neck: seven *cervical* vertebrae;
– in the back: twelve *thoracic* (dorsal) vertebrae, to which the ribs are attached;
– in the loin: five *lumbar* vertebrae;
– the rump-bone (*sacrum*): five *sacral* vertebrae, joined together in adults as a solid mass;
– the tail-bone (*coccyx*): four vertebrae, fused together.

The cervical, thoracic (dorsal) and lumbar vertebrae are separated from each other by thick pads of gristle (cartilage), known as the inter-vertebral discs, which allow movement of the spine and help to break the shock of any sudden force applied to the vertebral column (for example, when falling from a height on to the feet).

The whole spine is bound together by bands of strong fibrous tissue called ligaments.

Ribs and breastbone

The **ribs** consist of twelve pairs of curved bones extending from the thoracic vertebrae on either side round to the front of the body, the upper seven pairs being attached to the breastbone by cartilage. The next three pairs are attached by cartilage to ribs immediately above them. The last two pairs are unattached in front and are called 'floating' ribs.

The **breastbone** (*sternum*) is a dagger-shaped bone with the point downwards – (this point is just above the pit of the stomach).
The ribs and breastbone enclose and protect the lungs, the heart, major blood-vessels, the liver, stomach and spleen.

Shoulders and upper limbs

The bones of the shoulder are the collar-bone (*clavicle*) and the shoulder-blade (*scapula*).

The **collar-bone** can be felt between the upper part of the breastbone and the outer part of the shoulder. It is a narrow curved bone which forms a strut which supports and maintains the position of the upper limb away from the chest.

The **shoulder-blade** lies at the upper and outer part of

the back of the chest and forms joints with the collar-bone and the bone of the upper arm.

The upper limb comprises the upper arm, forearm, wrist and hand.

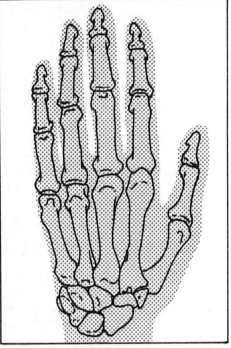

Figure 7: Articulated view of hand bones

The bone of the **upper arm** is the *humerus* which extends from the shoulder to the elbow, its upper and rounded head fitting into a shallow socket in the shoulder-blade. At its lower end it is connected with the bones of the forearm to form the elbow joint.

The two bones of the **forearm** are the *radius* on the outer or thumb side, and the *ulna* on the little finger side. They can rotate around one another and thus allow the turning of the hand. At the lower ends, the bones form the wrist joint with the *carpal* bones.

The **wrist** is composed of eight small carpal bones, arranged in two rows of four.

The palm of the **hand** has five long *metacarpal* bones, which also form the knuckles and support the short bones of the fingers and the thumb.

23

Each **finger** has three short bones (the *phalanges*), the thumb only two.

The **pelvis** is the large basin-like mass of bone attached to the lower part of the spine, being formed by the two **hip bones** and the *sacrum*. It supports the lower abdomen and protects its contents which include the bladder, the urethra and the lower part of the bowel and the back passage (*rectum*). In the female it also contains the womb (*uterus*) and the birth-canal (*vagina*). The pelvis also provides the deep sockets for the hip joints.

The **thigh-bone** (*femur*) extends from the hip to the knee and is the longest and strongest bone in the body. Its rounded head, supported on a neck, projects inwards to fit into the socket of the hip bone. At its lower end the thigh-bone forms part of the **knee-joint.**

The **knee-cap** (*patella*) is a small, flat, triangular bone lying in front of and protecting the knee joint.

The two bones of the **leg** are the *tibia* (shin-bone) and the *fibula*.

The tibia extends from the front of the knee to the ankle and forms part of the knee and ankle joints. Its sharp edges can be felt immediately below the skin of the front of the leg. The fibula lies on the outer side of the tibia and does

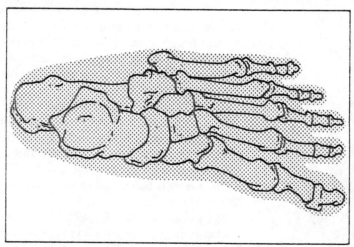

Figure 8: Articulated view of foot bones

24

not enter the formation of the knee-joint, but its lower end forms the outer part of the ankle-joint.

The **foot** is similar in many ways to the hand, and has the following bones:–
– seven irregular *tarsal* bones at the instep, the largest being the heel-bone while the uppermost forms the lower part of the ankle-joint;
– five long *metatarsal* bones in front of the instep supporting the bones of the toes;
– two short bones (the *phalanges*) in the big toe, and three in each of the other toes.

Joints

Joints are formed by the junction of two or more bones and are of two varieties:–

1. **Immovable** – where the edges of the bones are fitted firmly into each other so that the joint does not allow of movement. Such joints are to be found in the skull (*cranium*).

2. **Movable** – which are of three types:
(a) *Ball and Socket* joints, formed by the round head of one bone fitting into a cup-shaped cavity of another bone, thus allowing free movement in all directions. Examples: the shoulder and the hip joints.

(b) *Hinge* Joints, in which the surfaces of the bones are moulded to each other so as to allow free movement in one plane only, i.e. bending (flexion) and straightening (extension). Examples: the elbow and the knee joints.

(c) *Slightly movable* joints at which limited movement takes place. Examples: the wrist, the foot, between the vertebrae, and between the ribs and spine.

The ends of the bones of movable joints are covered with a smooth cartilage to minimise friction and are held together by bands of strong tissue (*ligaments*), the joint itself being enclosed by a lining of further strong tissue (the *capsule*). The inner lining (*synovial membrane*) of the capsule secretes fluid (*synovial fluid*) which acts as a lubricant.

Inside the knee-joint there are two pieces of cartilage (*semi-lunar*) which lie on the upper end of the tibia (shin-bone) and

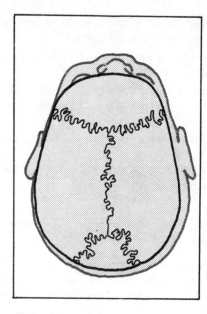

Figure 9: Immovable joint (skull)

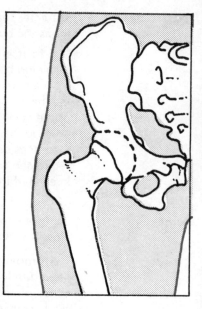

Figure 10: Ball and socket joint (hip)

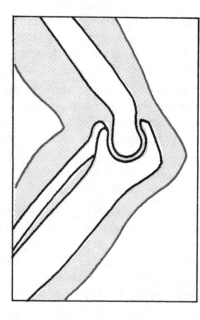

Figure 11: Hinge joint (elbow)

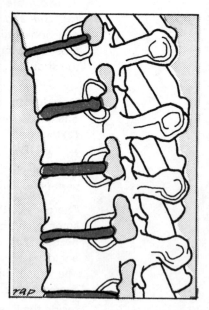

Figure 12: Slightly movable joint (spine)

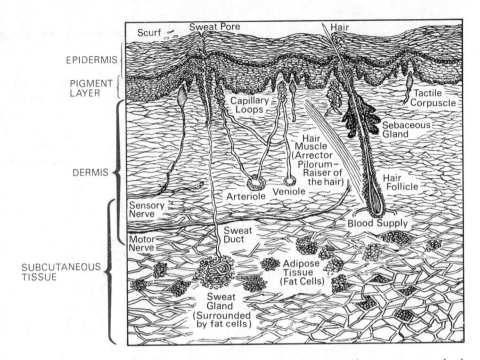

EPIDERMIS

PIGMENT LAYER

DERMIS

SUBCUTANEOUS TISSUE

Scurf — Sweat Pore — Hair

Capillary Loops

Hair Muscle (Arrector Pilorum – Raiser of the hair)

Arteriole — Veniole

Tactile Corpuscle

Sebaceous Gland

Hair Follicle

Sensory Nerve

Motor Nerve

Sweat Duct

Blood Supply

Adipose Tissue (Fat Cells)

Sweat Gland (Surrounded by fat cells)

Figure 13: Section of skin showing blood vessels, nerves, sweat glands and hair

deepen the surface for the rounded ends of the femur (thighbone).

Skin

This covers the whole of the body and protects underlying structures from injury and infection. Within it are numerous glands which secrete sweat, consisting mostly of water with a little salt (*sodium chloride*) and impurities from the blood. The sweat escapes through tiny openings on the surface of the skin (*pores*) where it evaporates and helps to regulate the temperature of the body.

Heat conservation

The layer of fat below the skin acts as an insulator and keeps in the heat produced in the deeper parts of the body. Loss of heat from the body is prevented when necessary by cutting down the flow of blood through the skin.

Dissipation of heat

The heat that is produced in the body through chemical processes and muscular contractions, as in exercise or

27

shivering, is dissipated largely by cooling of the blood flowing in the blood vessels of the skin.

Nerves

Sensory nerves carry all forms of sensation including pain, touch and temperature. All nerves are like white threads. Sensory nerves convey information to the spinal cord which then transfers it to the brain. If a sensory nerve is cut, the part of the skin supplied by it becomes numb.

Figure 14: Brain, spinal cord and nerves, showing examples of links to skin (sensory), to muscle (motor), and to organ (autonomic)

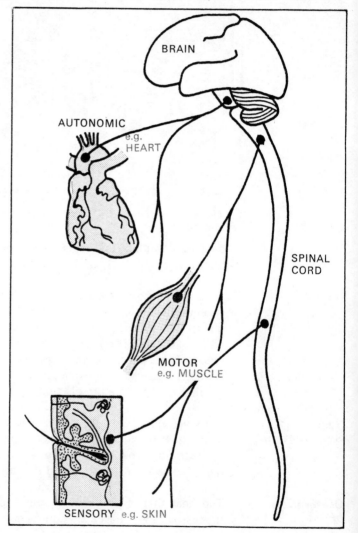

28

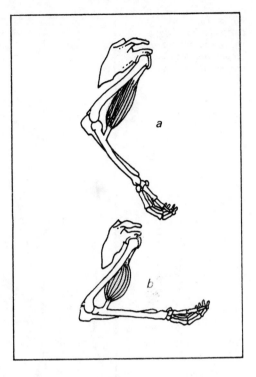

Muscles are activated and controlled by *motor nerves* which pass directly from the brain or by way of the spinal cord to the muscles. In this way the brain controls the activity of the body. If a motor nerve is cut or injured, the muscles or that group of muscles are paralysed.

A third set of nerves, the *autonomic system*, controls the heart, lungs, blood vessels, intestines, glands and other organs.

Muscles   These are to move various parts of the body and are of two types – voluntary and involuntary.

The **voluntary** muscles are controlled from the brain by motor nerves along which messages in the form of impulses are sent. Being under the control of the will, they produce movement as and when we wish. They are mostly attached to bone by strong bands (tendons) which run over joints.

29

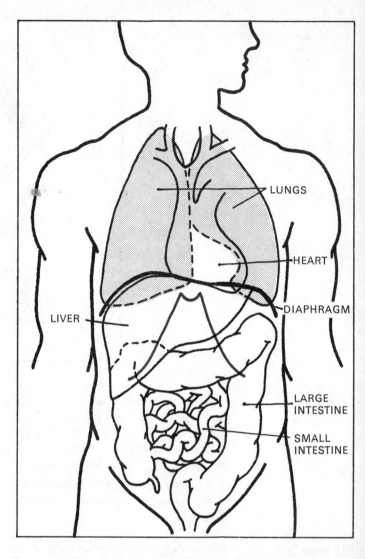

Figure 16: Trunk contents, front view, showing heart, lungs, diaphragm, liver, large and small intestine.

The muscles on getting shorter and thicker (contracting), provide the power to move bones.

The **involuntary** muscles are not under the control of the will, but continue to work at all times, even during sleep. They are to be found in the heart, and blood vessels, the walls of the stomach, the intestines (bowels) and in most of the internal organs.

30

*Figure 17: Trunk
contents, front view,
showing trachea,
œsophagus, stomach,
spleen, kidneys, ureters,
bladder*

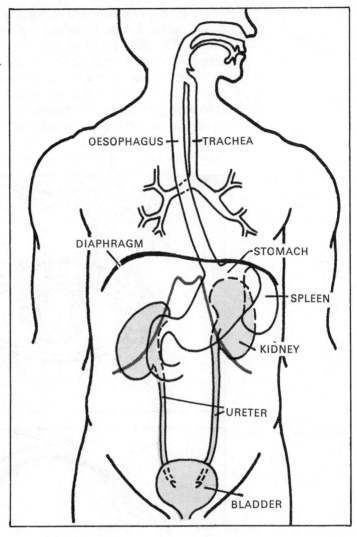

**Trunk and
contents**

The arched muscular partition (*diaphragm*) divides the trunk
into two cavities – the upper, the chest (*thorax*), the
lower (*abdomen*).

The upper cavity is bounded in front by the breastbone,
behind by the thoracic vertebrae of the spine, below by the
diaphragm, and is encircled by the ribs. It contains the
heart, the lungs, major blood vessels and the gullet.

The lower cavity is bounded above by the diaphragm, below by the pelvis, behind by the lumbar vertebrae and in front and at the sides by muscular walls. It contains several important organs – the **liver,** in the upper part of the abdomen covered mostly by the right lower ribs; the **spleen,** covered by the ribs on the upper part of the left side; the **stomach,** just below the diaphragm on the left side; the **pancreas,** behind the stomach; the **intestines,** which occupy the greater part of the cavity; the **kidneys,** at the back in the region of the loins; and the **bladder,** which lies

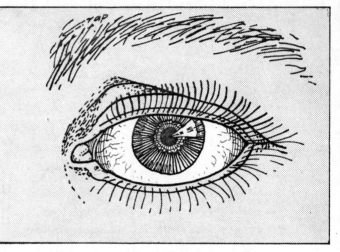

Figure 18: Eye, outer view

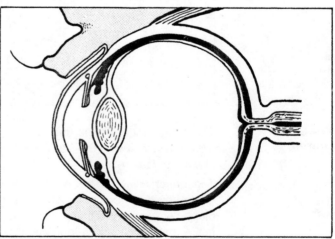

Figure 19: Eye, left side section

to the front of the. pelvis. Certain reproductive organs lie behind the bladder.

Eye

The eyes are situated in sockets in the front of the skull and are covered with folds of skin (the eyelids) from which the eyelashes project.

The inside of the eyelids and front of the eye are covered by a smooth membrane (*conjunctiva*) and are washed and kept moist by tear fluid.

Through the transparent part of the eye (*cornea*) can be seen a coloured circular diaphragm (the *iris*) with a round hole (the *pupil*). The latter varies in size with the amount of light passing through it.

Behind the pupil is the lens of the eye which focuses rays of light on to the light-sensitive part of the eye (*retina*).

Ear

The ear consists of three parts:

(*a*) The *outer ear* is that part which can be seen projecting from the side of the skull, together with the canal which leads to the eardrum.

(*b*) The *middle ear*, situated inside the skull, receives and transmits to the inner ear sound waves concerned in hearing. It also communicates with the back of the nose

Figure 20: The ear, cross-section, outer, middle and inner

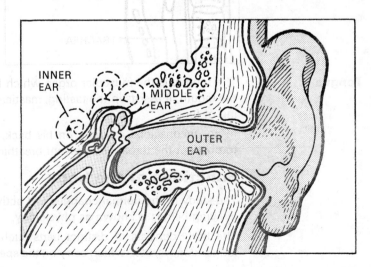

INNER
EAR

MIDDLE
EAR

OUTER
EAR

and throat by the Eustachian tube, which opens in swallowing.

(c) The *inner ear* is embedded inside the skull and is concerned with the sense of balance in addition to the sense of hearing.

The outer ear is separated from the middle ear by the eardrum.

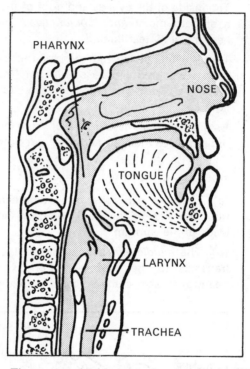

Figure 21: The nose, showing pharynx, the tongue, larynx and trachea

Tongue

The tongue is the muscular organ which lies on the floor of the mouth; it assists in the tasting, mastication and swallowing of food.

In an unconscious casualty on his back, the tongue tends to obstruct the throat and prevent breathing.

Functions of the body

The study of the normal changes and activities which go on in living beings is known as physiology.

The body consists of distinct parts such as the heart, the lungs, kidneys, etc., which carry on the special kinds of work.

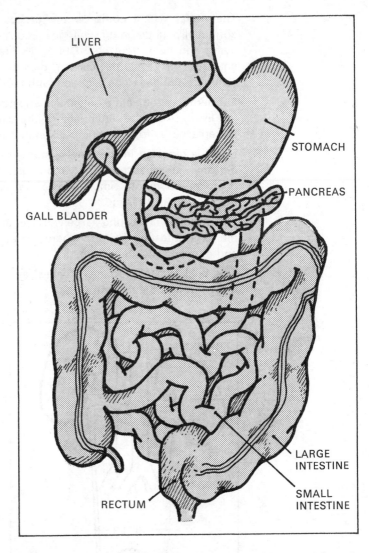

LIVER

STOMACH

PANCREAS

GALL BLADDER

LARGE
INTESTINE

SMALL
INTESTINE

RECTUM

Such a distinct part is called an 'organ' and its special work
is called a 'function'.

The essential functions of life such as respiration, circulation,
digestion, excretion, etc., are carried on by a set of organs
or closely related parts that form a 'system', e.g. the digestive
system which includes the mouth, the gullet, the stomach,
the liver, the pancreas and intestines.

35

The **cells,** which compose the tissues of the body, are continually undergoing changes and become worn out, dying and being replaced. During its life a cell undergoes change and gives off carbon dioxide and other waste products and has to be supplied with food and oxygen.

Furthermore, the various chemical substances that make up the living body are continually being used up and have to be replaced by food and fluid taken into the body.

Food is digested in the mouth, stomach and intestines, by digestive juices secreted by various glands and in this way is broken down into simple substances, which are absorbed from the small intestine.

The residue, consisting largely of vegetable fibres, enters the large intestine (*colon*) where the accompanying water and mineral salts are absorbed.

The final waste products (*faeces*) are eliminated from the body through the rectum.

*Figure 23:
Diagrammatic layout
of excretory (urinary)
system*

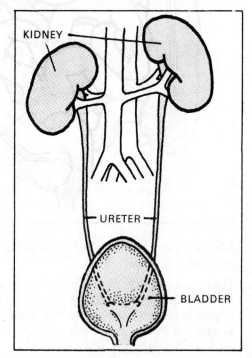

Oxygen is also necessary for the support of life and is obtained from the air we breathe. It must pass from the lungs into the blood stream and be circulated before it can be of use to the body. It unites with a protein in the red cells to form a suitable compound for easy transport throughout the body. Protein is a chemical compound which is derived from foodstuffs such as meat, eggs, fish etc.

The oxygen and the digested materials are carried in the blood stream to the tissues to supply substances for their growth and repair and to produce heat and energy.

Excretion – The soluble waste materials are carried away by the blood stream and removed through the lungs as carbon dioxide, through the kidneys as urine, through the glands in the skin as sweat. Insoluble (indigestible) waste products are also eliminated as faeces by the bowels.

Respiration

Respiration, or breathing, is the process by which oxygen passes from the air into the blood while carbon dioxide, a waste product, is expelled. This respiratory exchange of gases takes place in the lungs. Atmospheric air which we breathe comprises one fifth oxygen (20%) and four fifths nitrogen (80%).
There is still 16% oxygen in the air we breathe out. This accounts for the effectiveness of the expired-air method of resuscitation.

Lungs

The lungs occupy the greater part of the chest (*thoracic cavity*), one on each side of the heart. Their outer surfaces are covered with a membrane (*pleura*) which is continuous with the membrane lining the inner surfaces of the chest walls. These two layers move smoothly over each other as the lungs expand and relax during respiration.

Diaphragm

The diaphragm is a strong muscular partition separating the chest cavity from the abdominal cavity.

Airway

Air drawn into the lungs enters through the nose and mouth and passes down the throat (*pharynx*), through the voice box (*larynx*) to enter the windpipe (*trachea*). The top of the larynx is protected by a flap (*epiglottis*) which is open for breathing but shuts when food or fluid is being swallowed.

37

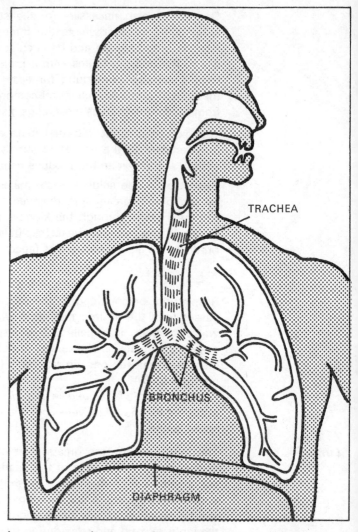

Figure 24: Lungs with trachea, bronchi and diaphragm

TRACHEA

BRONCHUS

DIAPHRAGM

In an unconscious casualty, the tongue may fall back and block the airway. The protective mechanism which prevents food or fluid from entering the larynx or windpipe does not operate if the casualty is unconscious. Accordingly it is vital in all unconscious casualties that a clear airway *must* be established *at once*.

In the chest the trachea divides into two branches, the right and left *bronchus*. Each bronchus passes into a lung

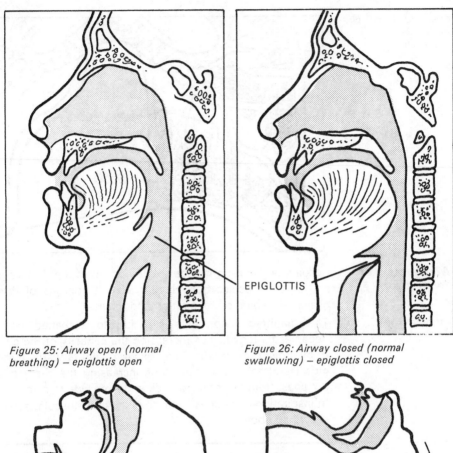

Figure 25: Airway open (normal breathing) – epiglottis open

Figure 26: Airway closed (normal swallowing) – epiglottis closed

EPIGLOTTIS

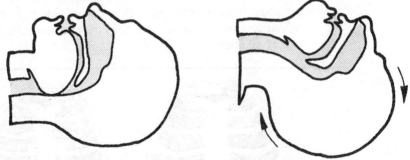

Figure 27 (left): Airway closed (unconscious) and (right) airway opened

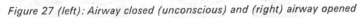

where it divides into a great number of small tubes (*bronchioles*), which, after repeated division into smaller and smaller tubes, open finally into numerous minute air-sacs (*alveoli*). A fine network of blood vessels (*capillaries*) surround the alveoli through which the exchange of gases takes place.

39

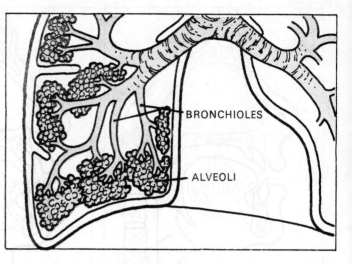

Mechanism of respiration

Respiration is brought about by the action of the diaphragm and of the muscles between the ribs. It consists of three phases – inspiration, expiration and a pause.

Inspiration

The diaphragm contracts and its dome-shaped centre becomes flattened, thus increasing the capacity of the chest from above downwards. The ribs are pulled upwards by the muscles attached to them, thus increasing the capacity of the chest from the front to back and from side to side.

In inspiration air is drawn into the lungs by muscular activity described above.

Figure 29: Inspiration
and expiration

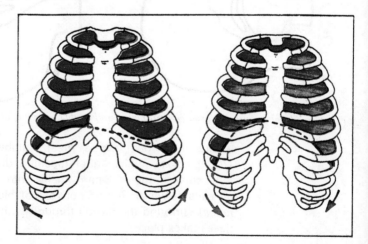

Expiration

In expiration, air is forced out through the bronchi and trachea by the relaxation of the diaphragm and the return of the ribs to their normal position. This is achieved by the elastic contraction of the lungs.

There is a short **pause** before inspiration re-commences.

These movements are controlled by respiratory centres in the mid brain which react to variation in the amount of carbon dioxide in the blood.

Rate of breathing

This may vary considerably. The average adult at rest breathes 15–18 times per minute. In infants and young children the respiration rate is 24–40 per minute.

The normal rate increases if more oxygen is required, as in exercise, fever or in conditions which affect the normal function of the lungs, e.g. pneumonia.

Blood and the circulation

Blood is continually circulated through the lungs and the body.

The liquid element of the blood is called *plasma*. It is a transparent yellow fluid in which are suspended the red and white corpuscles and platelets.

The **red corpuscles** are circular and biconcave in form, their red colour being due to a substance called *haemoglobin*. This substance forms a loose combination with oxygen and acts as the carrier of the oxygen in the blood, giving it its bright red colour. When the hæmoglobin has given off its oxygen to the tissues, the plasma takes up carbon dioxide and the colour of the blood changes to a darker shade of red.

The life of a red corpuscle is only a few weeks and they are continually being replaced by new ones from the red bone marrow. Normally there are 4–5 million red cells per cu. mm. of blood.

The **white corpuscles** are less numerous than the red and are constantly changing their shape. The larger ones are attracted to germs (*bacteria*) and quickly make their way out through the thin walls of the minute blood vessels (capillaries) into the surrounding tissues, to engulf and destroy them. If large numbers of these cells are killed

41

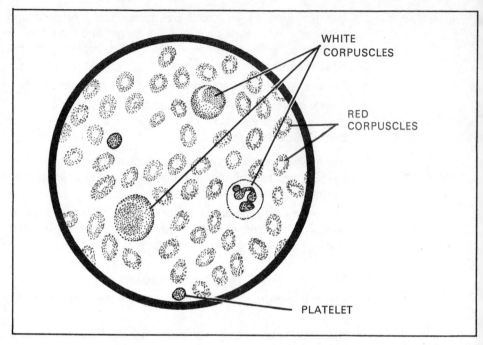

WHITE
CORPUSCLES

RED
CORPUSCLES

PLATELET

Figure 30: Blood film: red corpuscles, white corpuscles, platelets

by the germs, they, with the dead tissue of the cells, form pus. Normally there are 4000–8000 white corpuscles per cu. mm. of blood.

The **platelets** are developed from large white cells in the bone marrow and help in the clotting of blood.

The **blood** brings oxygen from the lungs and nutritive matter from the organs of the digestive system to the cells in the tissues of the body. It also carries away the soluble waste products of the tissue activity, to be got rid of through the lungs as carbon dioxide, through the kidneys as urine, through the glands as sweat.

The circulatory system

Blood vessels

The circulatory system consists of the *heart*, the *arteries*, the *capillaries* and the *veins*. The **heart** is the muscular organ which acts as a double pump. It lies in the chest behind the breast bone and rib cartilages, between the two lungs, and immediately above the diaphragm. The heart is divided into a right and left side, separated by a thin wall. Each side is further divided into an upper collecting chamber (*atrium*) and a lower thicker muscular pumping chamber (*ventricle*). Between each atrium and ventricle is a non-return valve, which allows the blood to flow in one direction only.

The **arteries** are the strongest of the blood vessels, their walls being strengthened by elastic and muscular tissue with a fibrous covering. They take the blood from the heart to all parts of the body. The arteries expand with the volume of blood forced along them by the pumping action of the heart, and then return to their normal size while the heart refills for the next contraction. Arteries continue to divide, becoming smaller and smaller until they become capillaries.

The **capillaries** are very small blood vessels, consisting only of a thin layer of cells which allow the exchange of fluids and gases to and from the tissue cells.

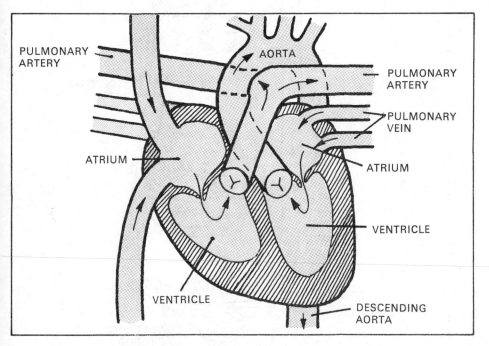

Figure 31: Heart and great vessels

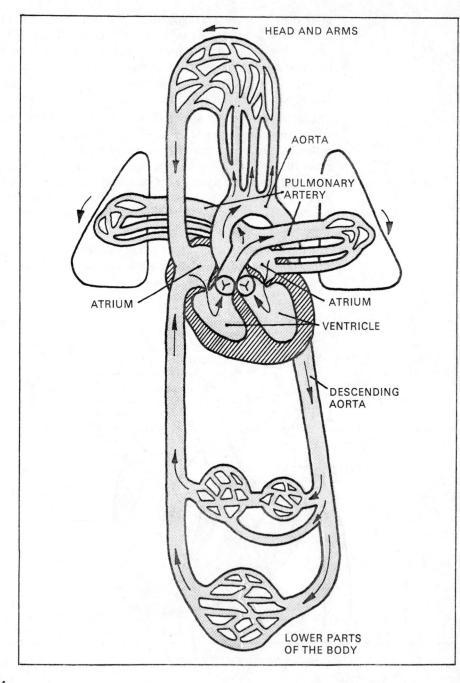

HEAD AND ARMS

AORTA

PULMONARY ARTERY

ATRIUM

ATRIUM

VENTRICLE

DESCENDING AORTA

LOWER PARTS OF THE BODY

The **veins** are formed by the joining up of the capillaries and take blood back to the heart. The smaller veins unite to form larger veins until they terminate in two main veins which enter the right collecting chamber (*atrium*) of the heart. The walls of the veins are thinner than those of the arteries and they have cup-like valves which allow the blood to flow only towards the heart.

Circulation of the blood

The right side of the heart pumps blood through the lungs — the *pulmonary* circulation.

The left side of the heart pumps this blood on throughout the body — the *systemic* circulation.

With each contraction of the heart, blood is forced from the ventricles through both of these circulatory systems, and with each relaxation of the heart, blood pours into the collecting chambers which then contract to fill the ventricles.

Pulmonary circulation

Venous blood, which has been collected by the two large veins, drains into the right collecting chamber (*atrium*) and from this chamber it passes through a valve into the right ventricle, which contracts and forces it through the pulmonary arteries to the lungs.

During its passage through the pulmonary capillaries, the blood gives off carbon dioxide and water vapour to be expired from the lungs and receives oxygen from the inspired air.

The blood, now rich in oxygen, returns in the pulmonary veins to the left collecting chamber of the heart from where it passes into the left ventricle.

Systemic circulation

The left ventricle contracts and forces oxygenated blood through the arteries.

The systemic circulation is the means by which the supply of oxygen, nutriment and fluid is distributed throughout the body and by which waste products are carried to the organs of excretion. The blood returns in the veins to the right atrium. The cycle is continuously repeated.

45

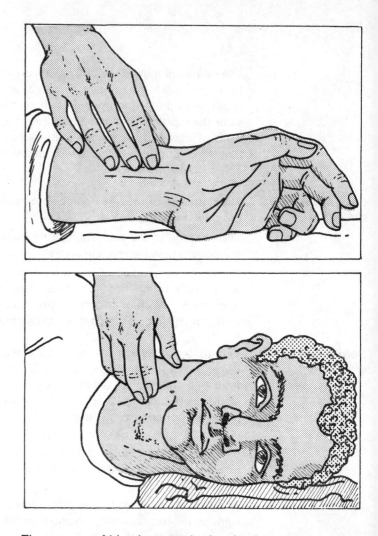

Figure 33: Taking radial pulse

Figure 34: Taking carotid pulse

Volume of blood   The amount of blood present in the circulatory system of an adult is approximately 10 pints (about 6 litres). When a large vessel is cut and blood escapes, the blood volume falls, the circulation fails, and the vital organs no longer receive adequate supplies of oxygen and nutriment.

Blood pressure   The pressure of blood in the arteries is largely determined by the force required to ensure that the blood reaches all parts of the body. This pressure becomes progressively less as the blood reaches the smaller arteries and capillaries.

Clotting of blood

When blood escapes from a damaged blood vessel it normally coagulates and forms a clot.

Pulse

The pulse beat is normally taken at the front of the wrist over the radial artery, about 1 cm in from the thumb side of the lower end of the forearm. The beat results from the thrust of blood at each contraction of the heart expanding the artery. The pulse may also be taken in many other suitable places.

The normal adult pulse rate at rest is 60–80 per minute, the average being 72.

In infants and young children, the normal resting rate is much higher; between 90 to 140 per minute.

Count the number of beats in thirty seconds and multiply by two. This gives the rate per minute. A watch with a seconds hand should be used to time the counting. Make a note of your findings.

Lymphatic system

As blood flows through the capillaries of the systemic circulation, fluid exudes through their walls, and bathes the cells of the body as it passes around them.

This fluid gives up its quota of oxygen, nutriment and water to the cells and takes in waste products including carbon dioxide. It then passes back into the blood stream through the capillaries (*lymphatics*).

There is also another system of hair-like tubes, called *lymph vessels*, which form a fine network throughout the body. These join up at intervals with small structures called the *lymphatic glands*, whose special function is to act as a barrier to germs which may enter the body. For example, when a person gets a septic finger, the glands in the arm-pit become swollen and tender as a result of their function of helping to prevent infection from getting into the general blood-stream with possible fatal result.

CHAPTER FOUR

Dressings and bandages

A dressing is a protective covering applied to a wound to –
- prevent infection;
- absorb discharge;
- control bleeding;
- avoid further injury.

The dressing itself must be germ free (*sterile*) if possible and act as a filter restricting the entry of germs (bacteria) which could cause infection of the wound.

It should also have a high degree of porosity. If sweat cannot evaporate through it, the skin becomes moist, the dressing sodden thus encouraging the growth of bacteria. Healing is assisted by keeping the wound and the surrounding skin dry.

A dressing helps blood to clot, which encourages healing to occur.

A non-adherent dressing, on removal, will not tear or damage the growing tissues (*granulations*) which repair the wound.

Adhesive dressings

These sterile dressings are of different kinds and consist of a pad of absorbent gauze or cellulose, with an adhesive backing which allows sweat to evaporate through it, if perforated.

The surrounding skin must be dry before application and all the edges of the dressing pressed firmly down.

Sterile adhesive dressings are supplied sealed in paper or plastic covers.

Non-adhesive dressings

Prepared (standard) Sterile Dressings: This sterile dressing consists of layers of gauze covered by a pad of cotton wool with an attached roller bandage to hold it in position. Only the bandage should be handled by the First Aider, who should quickly apply the dressing itself to the wound. The dressing is enclosed and sealed in protective coverings and is supplied in various sizes.

48

Figure 35: Standard dressing

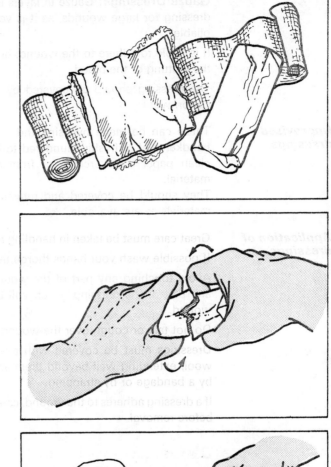

Figure 36: Standard dressing, opening

Figure 37: Standard dressing, application

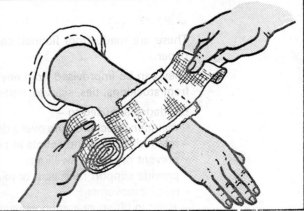

49

Gauze Dressings: Gauze in layers is commonly used as a dressing for large wounds, as it is very absorbent, soft and pliable.

It is liable to adhere to the wound; however, this may assist the clotting of the blood.

The dressing should be covered by one or more layers of cotton wool.

Improvised dressings

These can be made by using the inner surface of a clean handkerchief, a freshly laundered towel, a piece of linen, a clean paper handkerchief, or from other clean absorbent material.

They should be covered and retained in position by such materials as are available.

Application of dressings

Great care must be taken in handling and applying dressings.

If possible wash your hands thoroughly.

Avoid touching any part of the wound with the fingers, or any part of the dressing which will be in contact with the wound.

Do not talk or cough over the wound or the dressings.

Dressings must be covered with adequate pads of cotton wool, extending well beyond them and retained in position by a bandage or by strapping.

If a dressing adheres to the wound, careful soaking is required before removal.

Bandages

These are made from flannel, calico, elastic net or special paper.

They can be improvised from any of the above materials, or from stockings, ties, scarves, belts, etc.

Bandages are used to –
– maintain direct pressure over a dressing to control bleeding;
– retain dressings and splints in position;
– prevent or reduce swelling;
– provide support for a limb or joint;
– restrict movement;
– assist in lifting or carrying casualties.

Bandages should **not** be used for padding when other materials are available.

Unless bandages are applied firmly they are useless; dressings or splints will slip out of place, bleeding will not be controlled.

On the other hand, if a bandage is applied too tightly to a limb, it may injure the part or impede the circulation of the blood so that no pulse can be felt at the wrist or ankle.

A blueish tinge of the finger or toe nail beds may be a danger sign, as is loss of sensation.

Test for circulation

Press one of the casualty's nails of the bandaged limb so that it turns white. When pressure is released the nail bed should quickly become pink again, showing that the blood has returned. If it remains white or blue, or if the fingers are cold, the bandage is too tight.

Triangular bandage

The triangular bandage is made by cutting a piece of material (linen or calico) not less than one yard or one metre square, diagonally into two, thus producing two bandages.

Uses

As a whole cloth: In the form of a sling, or opened to its full extent for keeping a dressing in position.

As a broad bandage: The point is folded to meet the centre of the base and then the bandage is folded again in the same direction.

As a narrow bandage: Fold the broad bandage once again in the same direction.

As a ring pad: This may be made by passing one end of a narrow bandage once or twice round the finger, then bring the other end of the bandage through the loop and continue to pass it through and through until the whole of the bandage is used and a firm ring is made.

This pad may be used in the control of bleeding from a wound when a foreign body such as glass is present or an underlying fracture is suspected.

To tie a triangular bandage: The bandage should be tied with a reef knot, which does not slip and is flat and easy to untie.

The knot should be placed so that it does not cause discomfort by pressing on a bone, or chafe the skin at the back

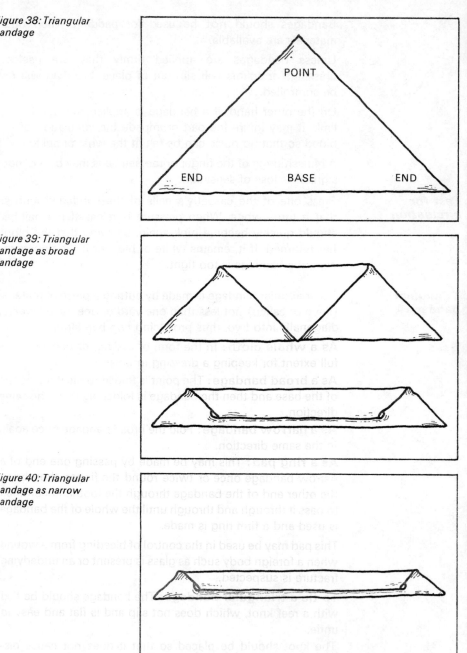

Figure 38: Triangular bandage

POINT

END BASE END

Figure 39: Triangular bandage as broad bandage

Figure 40: Triangular bandage as narrow bandage

52

of the neck when used on a sling. If the knot is uncomfortable, place some soft material beneath it as padding.

Remember when tying a reef knot, put:
1. Left over right, and
2. Right over left.
Tuck ends neatly away.

To pack the triangular bandages: When not in use, they should be folded narrow and the ends turned over towards the middle.

Slings

Slings are used when it is necessary to afford support and protection to the upper limb.

Arm sling
To support the forearm and hand where there are wounds and injuries of the upper limb and in some cases of fractured ribs. It is effective only when the casualty is sitting or standing.

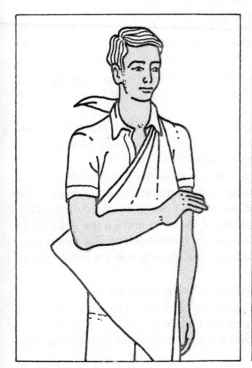

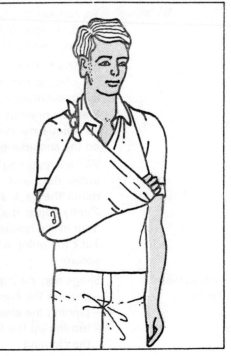

Figure 41: Arm sling *Figure 42: Arm sling*

Method: Support the forearm on the injured side, the wrist and hand a little higher than the elbow.

Place an open triangular bandage *between* the chest and the forearm, its point stretching well beyond the elbow.

Carry the upper end *over* the shoulder on the sound side, round the back of the neck to the front of the affected side.

Still supporting the forearm, carry the lower end of the bandage up over the hand and forearm and tie off in front of the hollow above the collar-bone. Bring the point forward and secure to the front of the bandage.

When an arm sling has been applied, the base of the bandage should be at the root of the little finger so that all finger nails are exposed for observation. If the circulation is impeded –

(a) the position of the hand should be altered;

(b) an adjustment made to the bandage; *or*

(c) the sling removed.

Triangular sling

To support the hand and forearm in a well-raised position as in the case of a hand injury, severely fractured ribs, or to provide additional support on a rough journey.

Method: The forearm on the injured side is supported across the chest with the fingers pointing towards the shoulder on the opposite side.

Place an open triangular bandage *over* the forearm and hand, its point extending well beyond the elbow, its upper end on the shoulder on the sound side.

While supporting the forearm, ease the base of the bandage under the hand, forearm and elbow; carry the lower end round the back and on to the front of the sound shoulder. Gently adjust the height of the sling and tie the ends off in front in the hollow above the collar-bone on the sound side. Tuck the point in between the forearm and the bandage and secure.

Improvised slings

Slings may be improvised in many ways, by –

– passing the hand inside the buttoned jacket or waistcoat;

– pinning the sleeve to the clothing;

– turning up the lower edges of the jacket and pinning it to the clothing;

– using scarves, belts, ties etc.

54

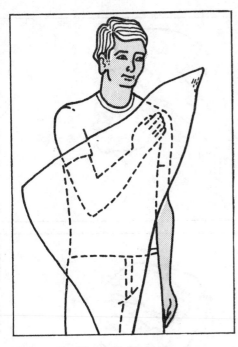

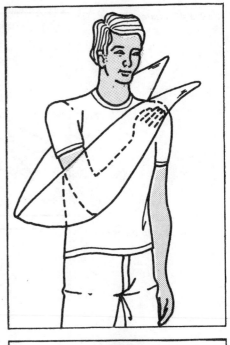

Figures 43, 44 and 45: Triangular sling

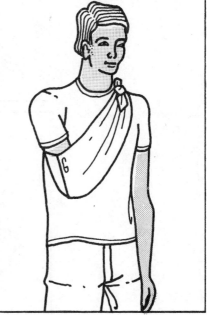

Figure 46: Scalp dressing

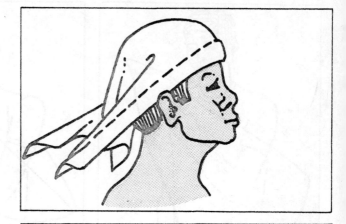

Figure 47: Scalp dressing

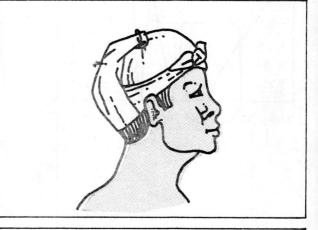

Figure 48: Scalp dressing (ring pad)

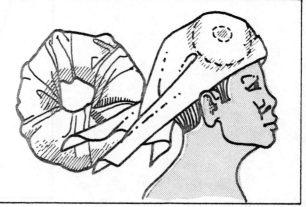

Application of triangular bandage

As a whole cloth to keep dressings in position: In the following applications of the triangular bandage, which is opened to its full extent, a narrow hem should be turned up along the inside of the base.

Scalp and head Stand behind the casualty and place the bandage so that the hem lies on the forehead close to the eyebrows and the point hangs down at the back of the head.

Carry the ends round the head just above the ears.

Cross the ends over the point of the bandage near the nape of the neck and bring them forward round the head above the ears.

Tie on the forehead close to the hem of the bandage.

Steady the head with one hand and with the other draw the point of the bandage downwards. Then turn it up and secure it to the bandage on the top of the head.

Chest (front) Stand in front of the casualty. Place the centre of the bandage over the dressing with the point on the shoulder of the same side. Carry the ends round the body and tie them, leaving one long end.

Carry the long end up and tie to the point on the shoulder.

Chest (back) Stand behind the casualty and proceed as for the front of the chest.

Shoulder, hip or groin Stand facing the injured side. In the case of the hip and groin, first tie a narrow bandage round the waist, knotting it on the injured side.

For the shoulder place a bandage over the shoulder with the point towards the ear.

For the hip or groin slip the point of a bandage under the knot of the narrow bandage round the waist.

Carry the hem of the bandage round the middle of the upper arm or thigh, cross the ends and tie on the outer side.

In the case of the shoulder, apply an arm sling.

Draw the point over the sling or narrow bandage and secure.

Elbow or knee Place the limb in a convenient position. Lay the point of the bandage on the back of the upper arm (front of thigh), the

57

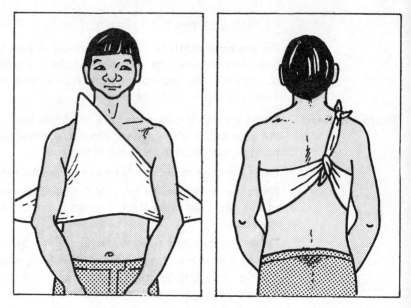

Figures 49 and 50: Bandaging the chest (front)

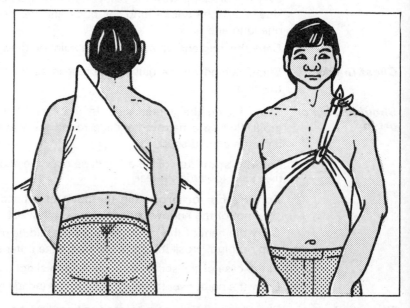

Figures 51 and 52: Bandaging the chest (back)

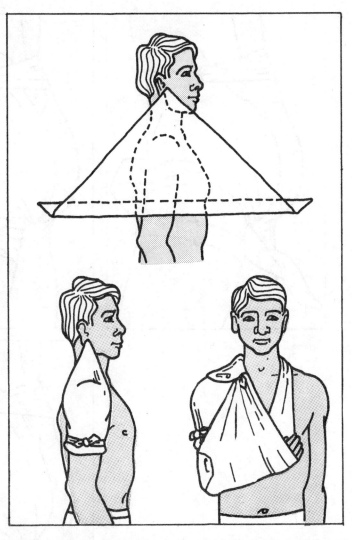

middle of its base lying in the back of the forearm (front of leg); cross the ends in front of the elbow (back of the knee) then round the arm (thigh) and tie above the joint. Finish off by bringing the point of the bandage over the knot and secure.

Hand, foot or stump   Pass an open bandage under the hand, foot or stump, with the point away from the casualty. Bring the point back on the

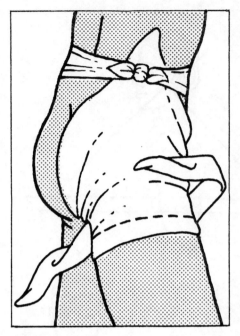

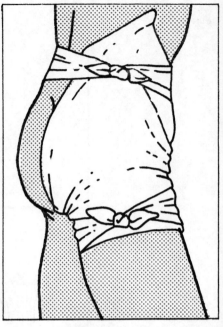

Figures 54, 55 and 56: Bandaging the hip

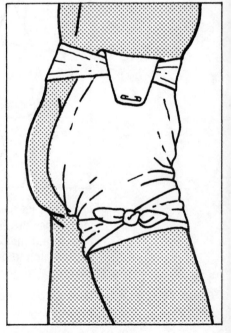

60

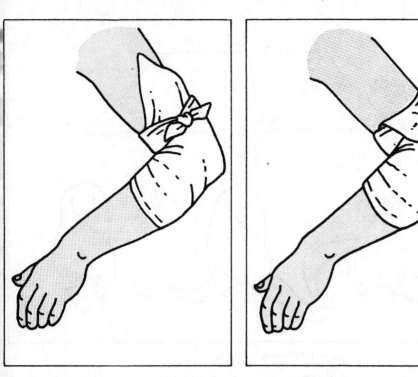

Figures 57 and 58:
Bandaging the elbow

hand, instep or stump. Pass the ends of the bandage round the wrist, ankle or stump, cross them and tie off over the

Figure 59: Bandaging
the foot

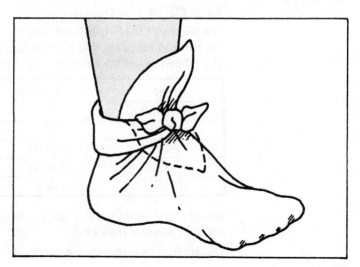

61

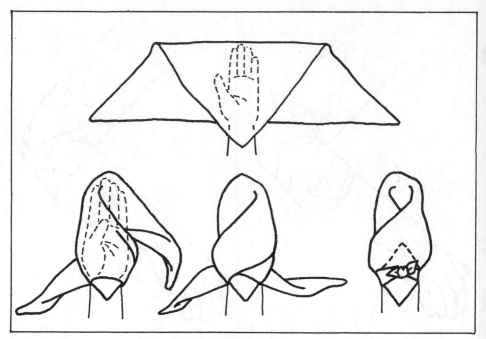

Figure 60: Bandaging the hand

point. Draw the point firmly downwards over the knot and secure.

The roller bandage

The widths of these bandages vary according to the parts of the body to be bandaged and the size of the casualty. The following are the average adult sizes:

Part	Width, inches	Width, cm.
FINGER	1	2·5
HAND	2	5
ARM	2 or 2½	5 or 6
LEG	3 or 3½	7·5 or 9
TRUNK	4 or 6	10 or 15

When partly unrolled, the roll is called the **head** and the unrolled part the **free end**.

The standard bandage is the rigid open weave type.

A 'conforming' bandage is more loosely woven, holds dressings lightly but firmly in place, even pressure being easily maintained.

Application

Rules for the application of roller bandages:

Use a tightly rolled bandage of suitable width.

Support the part to be bandaged. Stand in front of the casualty when bandaging an arm or leg. Bandage a limb in the position in which it is to remain. Hold the bandage with the head uppermost and apply the outer surface of the bandage to the part, unrolling only a few inches of the bandage at a time.

Bandage a limb from within outwards and from below upwards, maintaining even pressure throughout.

When bandaging a left limb the head of the bandage should be held in the right hand; when bandaging a right limb, in the left hand.

Begin the bandage with a firm oblique turn to fix it and allow each successive turn to cover two-thirds of the previous one, with the free edges lying parallel.

Finish off with a straight turn above the part, fold in the end and fasten with a safety pin, adhesive tape or bandage clip.

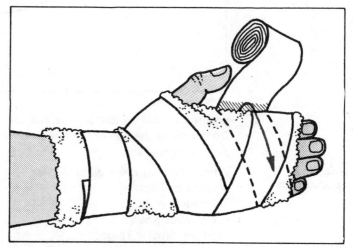

Figure 61: Roller bandage (hand)

63

Figure 62: Roller
bandage (forearm)

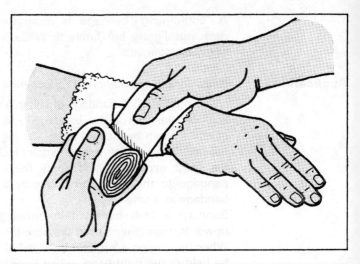

Figure 63: Roller
bandage (forearm)

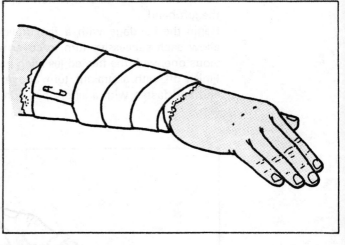

Ensure that the bandage is neither too tight nor too loose.
Do not cover the tips of the fingers or toes.
Test for circulation.

**Details of
application**

When applying roller bandages for –
– Hand or Foot;
– Forearm or Leg;
– Elbow or Knee;
– Upper Arm or Thigh;
the following details are as described for the upper limb

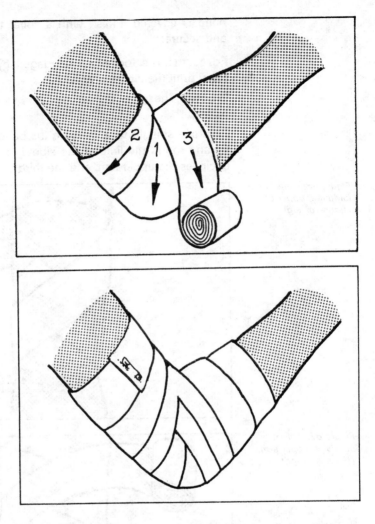

Figure 64: Roller bandage (elbow)

Figure 65: Roller bandage (elbow)

but are exactly the same in method for the lower limb.

Hand: *With the palm held downwards* – fix the bandage by a turn round the wrist and carry the roll obliquely over the back of the hand to the side of the little finger, then round the palm. Encircle the fingers with one horizontal turn so that the lower border of the bandage just reaches the root of the nail of the little finger. Carry the bandage back again round the palm and then return obliquely to the wrist; the figure of eight turns round the wrist and hand are repeated until the hand is covered. Finish with a spiral turn round the wrist and secure.

Forearm: The forearm is bandaged by use of the simple spiral until the elbow is reached.

Elbow: The joint should be bandaged in a comfortable position.

Take one straight turn, carrying the bandage over the elbow tip and round the limb at the elbow level. The second turn encircles the upper arm, and the third turn the forearm, each

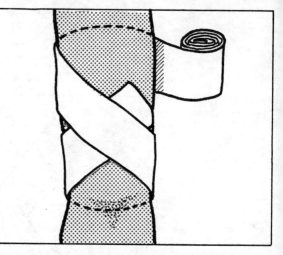

Figure 66: Roller bandage, upper arm (figure-of-eight)

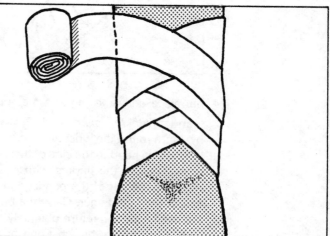

Figure 67: Roller bandage, upper arm (figure-of-eight)

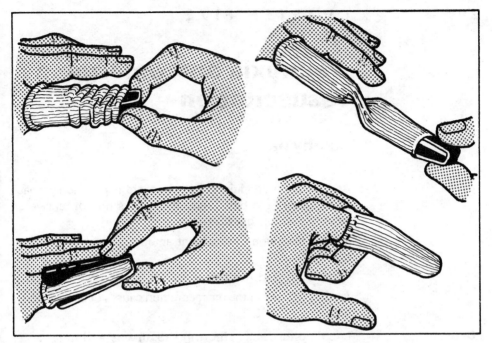

Figure 68: Tubular gauze bandage

being made to cover the margins of the first turn.

Continue the turns alternately above and below the first turn allowing each to cover a little more than two-thirds of the previous turn. Finish above the elbow.

Upper Arm: This is bandaged by a succession of simple spiral or figure-of-eight turns and the bandage may be carried on from the forearm or elbow or started independently, as convenient.

Tubular gauze bandage

This is a method of bandaging which is in many ways better and quicker than traditional methods, but is more expensive. It consists of a roll of seamless tubular gauze in various sizes to fit different parts of the body. It is applied with specially designed applicators.

Elasticised net bandage

Elasticised net bandage, a two-way stretch mesh material, is easy to apply, and comfortable to wear; it can be used on the head, the trunk or the limbs.

67

CHAPTER FIVE

Asphyxia and emergency resuscitation

Asphyxia

Asphyxia is a condition in which there is commonly a lack of oxygen in the blood, and the tissues do not receive an adequate supply because —

— there may be an insufficient amount of oxygen in the air breathed, *or*

— the lungs and heart have ceased to function effectively.

Asphyxia is one of the most common causes of unconsciousness.

Causes

Local conditions affecting the airway and lungs:—

Spasm caused by —
— *Food,* 'down the wrong way';
— *Water,* as in some instances of drowning;
— *Smoke,* bronchitis, hiccups, irritant gases, asthma.

These may cause severe spasms of some part of the respiratory tract, preventing the passage of air.

Obstruction caused by —
— the tongue falling to the back of the throat in an unconscious casualty lying on his back or in the case of a fractured jaw;
— a mass of food;
— a foreign body such as teeth, blood, vomit;
— swelling of the tissues of the throat due to injury such as in stings, scaldings; swallowing of corrosives or following infection.

Suffocation by pillows, plastic bags etc.

Compression of the neck caused by —
— tie, collar, stocking or scarf in strangulation;
— hanging, throttling.

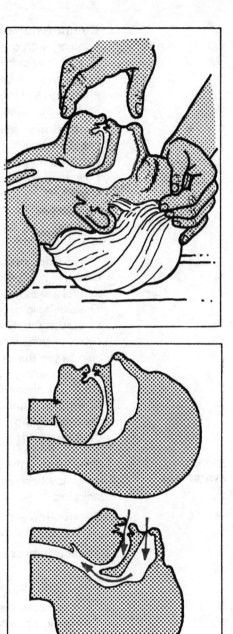

Figure 69: Extending the head to ensure airway

Figure 70: Cross-section of closed and open airway (unconscious)

69

Compression of the chest caused by –
– fall of earth or sand, compression by grain in silo;
– crushing against a wall or barrier;
– pressure in a crowd;
– damage to lung as a result of a sucking wound, or 'stove-in' chest, common in motor accidents.

Conditions affecting the nerves which control respiration:
Electrical injury;
Poisoning – barbiturates, morphia, industrial gases, pesticides;
Muscle contractions – as in tetanus (lockjaw);
Paralysis – as in apoplexy and in some nerve illnesses such as poliomyelitis; or in injury to spinal cord.

Conditions preventing the use of oxygen by the body:
Carbon monoxide poisoning – household gas (except natural gas as from the North Sea) and motor exhaust fumes. The available oxygen in the blood is progressively replaced by carbon monoxide.
Cyanide poisoning (prussic acid gas): The tissues are unable to use the oxygen present in the blood.
Air containing insufficient oxygen (e.g. smoke-laden buildings, disused shafts, tunnels).
Change in atmospheric pressure (e.g. high altitudes and deep sea diving).
Continuous fits preventing adequate breathing.

Signs and symptoms

Breathing – the rate, depth and difficulty increase at first; later may become noisy with frothing at the mouth, finally stopping.

Congestion – of the head and neck, face, lips, conjunctivae and nail beds of fingers and toes may become blue (cyanosis).

Consciousness is gradually lost; fits may occur.

Emergency resuscitation

The vital needs are –
– **Airway**: open to allow air to reach the lungs;
– **Breathing**: adequate to allow sufficient oxygen to enter the lungs and pass into the blood.;
– **Circulation**: sufficient to carry the oxygen-containing

blood to the tissues of the body.

It is essential for the brain to be continuously supplied with oxygenated blood; if totally deprived of oxygen for more than about four minutes, it is likely to be permanently damaged: some of this time may already have elapsed. It may, in fact, be possible to resuscitate such a casualty but his subsequent mentality may be affected.

Emergency resuscitation is therefore concerned with –
– the immediate and continued oxygenation of the blood by inflating the lungs;
– the restarting of the heart to maintain sufficient circulation to ensure that this oxygenated blood reaches the brain and other organs (e.g. heart, kidney).

The most important single factor in any form of respiratory resuscitation is the speed with which the first few inflations can be given.

When artificial respiration is necessary, the urgency is so great that only obvious obstructions should be moved –
– *over the head and face:* plastic bag, pillow;
– *round the neck:* constriction as in strangulation;
– *in the mouth:* debris, vomit, blood, loose teeth or tongue.

It is important to realise that First Aid measures may have to

Figure 71: Clearing the mouth of debris

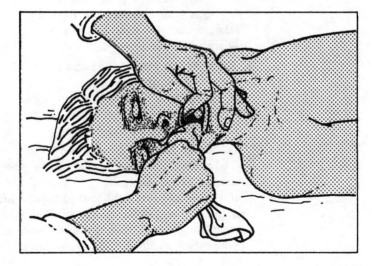

be continued until the casualty reaches hospital.

Respiratory resuscitation (artificial respiration)

There are several methods of artificial respiration.
The *most effective* is mouth-to-mouth (mouth-to-nose) and this method can be used by almost all age groups and in almost all circumstances *except* –
– when there is severe injury to the face and mouth;
– when the casualty is pinned in the face down position;
– if vomiting interferes with respiratory resuscitation.
Vomiting usually occurs when breathing is re-established and consciousness is returning.

A person who is asphyxiated to any significant degree will be in a state of unconsciousness.
In this state, however brought about, the casualty is likely to die – simply because his tongue may have fallen to the back of his throat and blocked his airway. This obstruction may be aggravated by vomit or other matter.
The first thing to do therefore with an unconscious casualty is – to check that he is breathing easily. If he is NOT, then the following treatment should be carried out immediately.
Waste no time. Start emergency resuscitation immediately. Seconds count.

Treatment

If the casualty is NOT breathing –
1. Ensure he has a good airway –
– support the nape of the neck and press the top of the head so that it is tilted backwards;
– push the chin upwards.

These moves extend the head and neck and lift the tongue forward clear of the airway.
If the casualty is capable of breathing, this may be all that is necessary; he will gasp and start to breathe. At this point, place him in the recovery position.

2. Loosen clothing at neck and waist;
3. To help his breathing, three or four inflations of the lungs may be useful.
If the casualty does not start to breathe after having ensured a good airway, keep the head tilted backwards and begin mouth-to-mouth (to-nose) breathing; this is easier to do when the casualty is lying on his back.

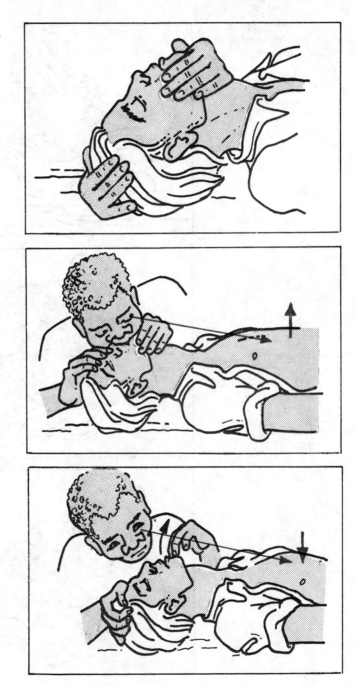

Figures 72, 73 and 74:
Mouth-to-mouth method
of artificial respiration

Figures 75, 76 and 77:
Mouth-to-nose method of
artificial respiration

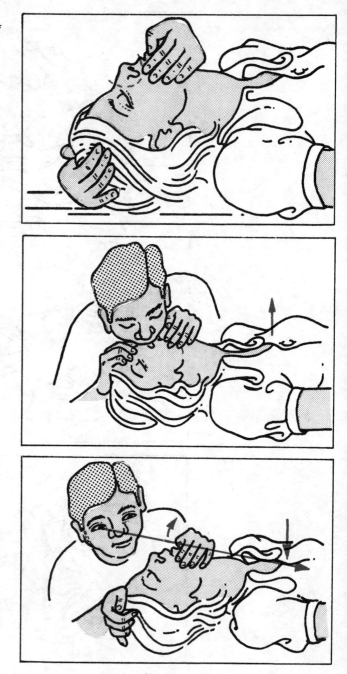

In an adult –
– open your mouth wide and take a deep breath;
– pinch the casualty's nostrils together with your fingers;
– seal your lips round his mouth;
– blow into his lungs until the chest rises;
– then remove your mouth, and watch the chest fall;
– repeat and continue inflations at your natural rate of breathing.

In an infant or young child –
– open your mouth wide and take a deep breath;
– seal your lips round his mouth and nose;
– blow *gently* into his lungs until the chest rises;
– then remove your mouth and watch the chest fall;
– repeat and continue inflations.

Give the first four inflations as rapidly as possible to saturate the blood with oxygen.

If the casualty's chest fails to rise, there is an obstruction. Ensure that his head is tilted well backwards; turn him on his side and thump his back. Check for and remove any foreign matter from the back of the throat.

It may be easier to obtain an airtight seal between your mouth and that of the casualty if his dentures are retained securely in their normal position. If the First Aider cannot make a seal round the casualty's mouth, he should use the mouth-to-nose method. In this case, during inflation, the casualty's mouth should be closed with the thumb of the hand holding the lower jaw.

If the heart is beating normally continue to give artificial respiration until natural breathing is restored; send for ambulance after placing him in the recovery position.

If the heart is NOT beating – as shown by the following –
– the casualty's colour remains or becomes blue/grey;
– the pupils are widely dilated when visible;
– the carotid pulse cannot be felt.
1. Put him on his back on a firm surface – the floor.
2. Strike his chest smartly to the left of the lower part of the breastbone with the edge of the hand; this may re-start the heart beating.

75

3. If no response at first to this stroke, start external heart compression at once.

Remember: In *respiratory arrest* it is safe and wise to commence artificial respiration while breathing appears to be failing.

In *cardiac arrest* external heart compression should **not** be started unless you are satisfied that the heart has stopped beating.

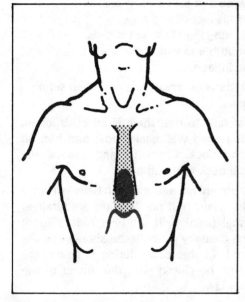

Figure 78a: Position of sternum.

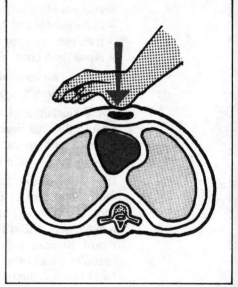

Figure 78b: Cross-section through chest.

External heart compression

Method—
1. Place yourself at the side of the casualty;
2. Feel for the lower half of the breastbone;
3. Place the heel of your hand on this part of the bone, keeping the palm and fingers off the chest;
4. Cover this hand with the heel of the other hand;
5. With arms straight, rock forwards pressing down on the lower half of the breastbone (in an unconscious adult it can be pressed towards the spine for about one and a half inches (4 cm)).

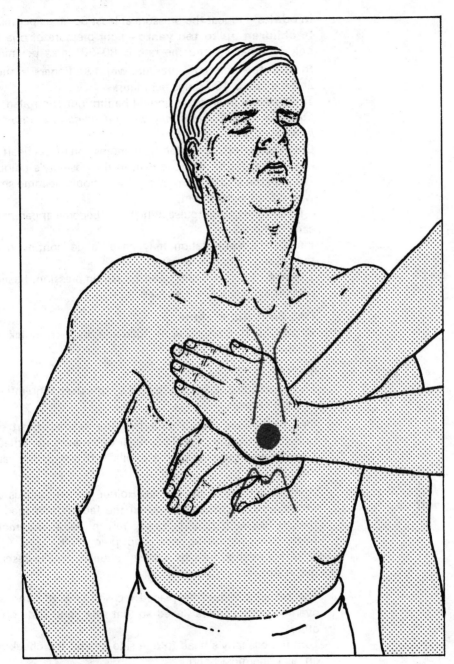

Figure 78c: External heart compression.

In adults – repeat the pressure at least 60 times per minute

In children up to ten years – light pressure of one hand only is sufficient and the rate is 80–90 times per minute

In infants – very light pressure with two fingers is enough and the rate is 100 times per minute.

The pressure in all cases should be firm but controlled.

Erratic or violent action may cause damage to the ribs or to internal organs.

Check the effectiveness of the compression of the heart by –

– watching for an improvement in the casualty's colour;

– noting the size of the pupils, which should become smaller with effective treatment;

– feeling the carotid pulse, which will become apparent with each compression.

Emergency resuscitation may have to be continued until the casualty reaches hospital.

The rate of lung inflation and heart compression, based on present experience, are as follows: –

One First Aider alone

FIVE Fifteen heart compressions followed by two quick lung inflations and then repeat.

Two First Aiders

Five heart compressions followed by one deep lung inflation and then repeat.

One First Aider should undertake the external heart compression while the other First Aider undertakes the inflations (also noting the size of the pupils and feeling for carotid pulsation).

Holger Nielsen method

Another method is the revised Holger Nielsen, and is used in certain circumstances – when the face is damaged and the jaw has been fractured or severely injured so that mouth-to-mouth or mouth-to-nose is not practicable.

A further method for use in these circumstances is described in the Appendix. (Silvester).

The casualty should be placed face downwards, the arms overhead, the elbows flexed so that one hand rests on the other.

Turn the casualty's head to one side so that the cheek rests on his uppermost hand.

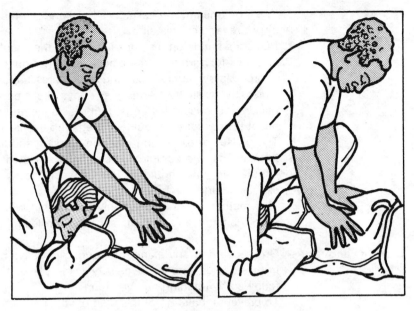

Figures 79 and 80: Holger Nielsen method of artificial respiration

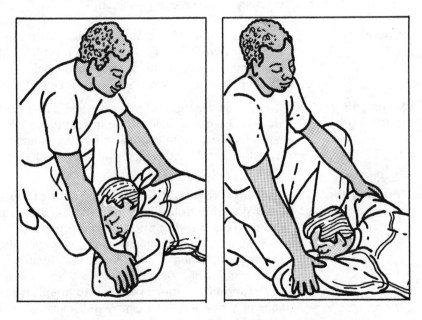

Figures 81 and 82: Holger Nielsen method of artificial respiration

Kneel on one knee at casualty's head and put the foot of the opposite leg near his elbow.

Place the hands on his back just below the shoulder blades, and rock forward with the elbows straight until the arms are approximately vertical, exerting steady pressure on his chest. Grasp the casualty's arms just above the elbow and rock backwards, raising his arms until resistance and tension are felt at the casualty's shoulders, then drop the casualty's arms. The phases of expansion and compression should each last $2\frac{1}{2}$ seconds, the complete cycle being repeated 12 times a minute. No time should be lost between the two phases of expansion and compression.

This method is, of course, only practicable when there are no gross injuries to the arm, shoulder-girdle and ribs.

During recovery

On recovery at any stage, outpouring of saliva and of fluid from stomach and nose usually takes place; this may be followed by retching and vomiting.

To prevent inhalation of this fluid or vomit, which may cause subsequent infection of the lungs, place the casualty carefully in the recovery position.

Drowning

A large number of deaths are caused by drowning every year. When fresh water is breathed into the lungs it is largely absorbed, but sea water is less well absorbed. Sometimes spasm of the larynx may prevent water entering the lungs.

Signs and symptoms

The face and particularly the lips and ears of the casualty are congested and may be livid in colour.

A fine foam-like froth may exude from his mouth and nostrils. It is this froth in the small airways of the lungs which obstructs the passage of air.

Treatment

The aim is to get air into the casualty's lungs with the least possible delay and then, if necessary, to ensure the heart is beating and blood circulating.

1. Start resuscitation immediately, quickly removing any obvious obstructions from the casualty's mouth.

2. Continue while wading ashore with the casualty.

3. **Arrange for urgent removal to hospital** as complications may develop, for example, inflammation and swelling (œdema) of the lungs.

Poisoning by carbon monoxide	Apart from deliberate self-administration, poisoning occurs by accident in the aged owing to faulty memory and diminishing sense of smell or hearing, through defective household gas appliances, coke stoves and cracked pipes of flues. The inhalation of fumes from the partial combustion of fuel or other material and from motor exhausts also constitutes a danger.
Signs and symptoms	Carbon monoxide poisoning can cause impairment of judgement and obstructive unco-operative behaviour. The casualty may be found – – confused, stuporous or in a coma.
Action	The use of a life-line when entering a gas filled room or space is a safety precaution which should be used whenever available. If the casualty is in a room or enclosed space, before entering breathe in and out several times and then take a deep breath and hold it. Go in and get the casualty out. If you cannot do so at once, cut off the source of danger – turn off the gas; switch off the engine; obtain a full supply of fresh air; open doors and windows *and get out.*
Treatment	If breathing is failing or has stopped, start resuscitation immediately. After rescue, ensure absolute rest, placing the casualty in the recovery position.
Poisoning by carbon dioxide	May cause collapse in those working over vats in breweries and in deep wells or sewers.
Treatment	As for poisoning by carbon monoxide.
Suffocation by smoke	Protect yourself by tying a towel or coarse cloth, preferably wet, over your mouth and nose. The use of a life-line is a safety precaution and should be used whenever available: **Keep low and remove the casualty as quickly as possible** In smouldering hazards, care must be taken not to increase the fire risk by leaving doors and windows open.
Treatment	As for poisoning by carbon monoxide.

Figure 83: Removal of obstruction – infant

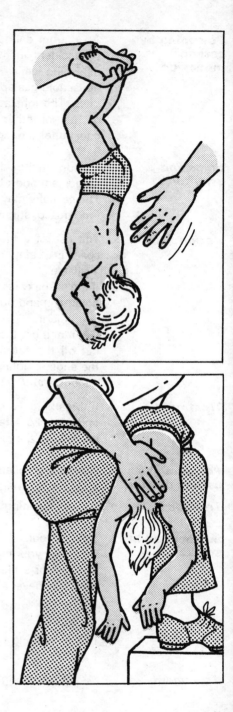

Figure 84: Removal of obstruction – child

Choking

A common incident at all ages. The obstruction to breathing is largely due to spasm.

Signs and symptoms

The casualty may or may not have a fit of coughing. His face and neck are congested and may become livid. Violent and alarming attempts at inspiration may be made.

Treatment

The aim of First Aid is to remove any foreign body and relieve the spasm or, if necessary, to get air to the lungs past the foreign body if this cannot be removed.

Remove any obvious obstruction—a lump of food, false teeth. If the obstruction is thought to be in the windpipe, in the case of —

An infant
– hold the infant up by the legs;
– smack him smartly three or four times between the shoulders. This should dislodge any foreign body;
– give artificial respiration, if necessary.

A child
– lay the child over your knee, head downwards;
– give three or four sharp slaps between the shoulders to dislodge the obstruction.
– give artificial respiration, if necessary.

An adult
Immediately strike him three or four sharp blows between the shoulders;
After clearing any obstruction from the throat, give artificial respiration, if necessary.

Hanging, strangulation, throttling

These conditions commonly occur accidentally: due to lack of air (oxygen) there is a failure of respiration.

Signs and symptoms

Similar to those of severe asphyxia.

Treatment

1. Remove the cause or relieve the obstruction –
– tear open the plastic bag;
– if the casualty is suspended, raise him;
– loosen the cause of obstruction.
2. If necessary give artificial respiration.

Electrical injury

Injury is the result of passage of an electrical current through the body. The immediate effect may be extremely severe and cause irregular quivering or tremor of muscles of the heart (*fibrillation*) or stop its action with cessation of breathing.

High voltage injuries

Electric current up to 400,000 volts *from overhead electric cables, conductor rails of electric railways and some industrial currents.*

Contacts with electric currents of such high voltage may be immediately fatal, or cause some serious injury, including severe burns.

Sudden muscle spasm may throw the casualty with some force away from the point of contact and further injuries, such as broken bones, may result. If this occurs, the casualty should be treated in accordance with the priorities of his injuries. When spasm affects the muscles of the chest, asphyxia may result.

Should the casualty remain in contact with, or in close proximity to, such a high voltage electric current, *no attempt at rescue must be made.*

Do not allow anyone within twenty yards. Get someone to contact the police. No safe approach to render first aid can be made until you are absolutely sure that:—
– the cable or conductor rail is out of service;
– it is isolated and earthed near the site of the accident, as it may at any moment, without warning, be re-energised.

Insulating material such as dry wood, clothing etc. is not proof against these high voltages which can jump a considerable gap, so also causing flash burns.

NEVER climb an electric pylon or pole in anticipation of rendering first aid.

Cranes and other tall objects sometimes foul overhead electric lines. If they remain in contact with or in close proximity to the line, no approach should be made until it has been established that it is safe to do so.

When you are officially informed that it is safe, render first aid.

Low voltage injuries

Electricity current of low voltage *from the domestic supply*

It should be realised that moisture and water conduct electricity, and accordingly it should be carefully noted that when the switches are faulty and an attempt is to be made to carry out the rescue of a person who is in contact with an electrical current, care must be taken to avoid direct contact with the casualty, thus preventing injury to yourself.

Injury may stop the action of the heart and of breathing.
The local effect is a burn which is deeper than its size suggests.

Action   Break the contact – switch the current off; remove the plug; wrench the cable free. If this is impossible, stand on some dry insulating material and by means of dry wood, folded newspaper or rubber, attempt to break the contact, for example, by pushing the casualty's limbs away. Do not touch the casualty with your hands.

Treatment   If necessary give artificial respiration; treat burns.

Lightning injury   Lightning may produce similar injuries to those of a high voltage electric current.

Instantaneous death may occur. On being struck by lightning, the casualty is stunned and falls unconscious to the ground. There may be patches of scorching on the skin, burns being deeper where a metallic object, such as a watch, has been carried close to the skin.
Clothing may be set on fire.

Treatment   If necessary give artificial respiration; treat burns.

85

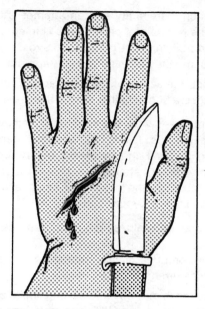

Figure 85: Incised wound

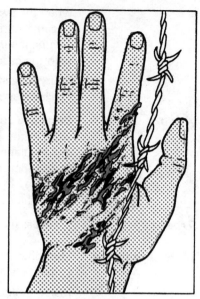

Figure 86: Lacerated wound

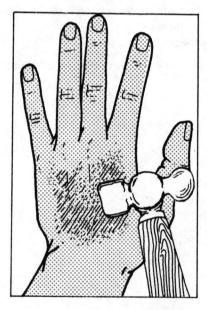

Figure 87: Contused wound

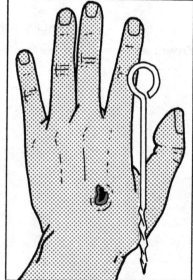

Figure 88: Punctured wound

CHAPTER SIX

Wounds, bleeding and circulatory failure

A wound is an abnormal break in the continuity of the tissue of the body which permits the escape of blood, externally or internally, and may allow the entrance of germs causing infection.

Wounds may be classified as follows:

1. **Incised or clean cut** caused by a sharp instrument such as a knife or razor. They may bleed profusely.

2. **Lacerated or torn** caused by such things as machinery, claws of an animal or barbed wire. The edges of the wound are torn and irregular and usually bleed less freely than incised wounds. Dirt is more likely to be present.

3. **Contused or bruised** caused by a blow from a blunt instrument, fall against a hard surface or by crushing.

4. **Punctured or stab** caused by a sharp pointed instrument such as a dagger, garden fork, stiletto, needle etc. These wounds have comparatively small openings but may be deep, causing serious injury.

5. **Gunshot wounds.** A small entry may be associated with extensive internal injuries and with a large exit wound.

Bleeding

Bleeding may occur externally or internally and may vary from trivial to severe or fatal.

The body possesses certain built-in mechanisms that tend to stop bleeding spontaneously, and it is important to realise this. For example:-

(a) Shed blood will clot, so tending to block the damaged vessel;

87

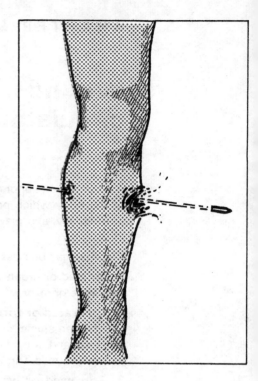

Figure 89: Gunshot wound: small entry, larger exit

(*b*) The cut ends of a blood vessel will contract, thus diminishing the loss of blood;

(*c*) The blood pressure falls and there is consequently less force to push blood out of the vessel;

(*d*) The skin vessels constrict and reduce bleeding.

Signs and symptoms

As the result of severe loss of blood, *external or internal,* the following occurs:—

— face and lips become pale;

— skin cold and clammy;

— casualty feels faint or dizzy;

— pulse rapid, becoming weaker;

— restlessness; casualty complains of thirst;

— complains of feeling sick;

— breathing becomes shallow, sometimes accompanied by yawning and sighing: casualty may gasp for more air ('air hunger').

These signs and symptoms may vary widely in different

persons and in different circumstances and with the rate of bleeding.

External bleeding

Wounds with slight bleeding: Blood may ooze from all parts of the wound and may appear alarming, but the bleeding usually stops of its own accord. It is easily controlled by local pressure.

Treatment

1. Reassure casualty;
2. Place him at rest;
3. Apply a dressing with a pad if necessary and bandage firmly in position. An adhesive dressing may be suitable;
4. Raise the injured part and support it in position, unless an underlying fracture is suspected;
5. If the wound is dirty, before applying the dressing, if possible, wash the wound with running water from the middle outwards. Temporarily protect the wound with a sterile swab and gently clean the surrounding skin. Dry the skin with swabs of cotton wool, wiping away from the wound and using each swab only once.

Wounds with severe bleeding

Treatment

The aim of First Aid is to stop the bleeding immediately and to obtain medical aid urgently.

1. Apply direct pressure with the fingers to the bleeding point or points, over a dressing if immediately available, for 5–15 minutes. If the wound area is large, press the sides of the wound firmly but gently together.
2. Lay the casualty down in a suitable and comfortable position, and lower the head if possible.
3. Raise the injured part and support it in position, unless an underlying fracture is suspected.
4. Carefully remove from the wound any foreign bodies which are visible and can easily be picked out or wiped off with a dressing.
5. When a dressing is available —
   – apply it directly over the wound and press it firmly down;
   – cover it with a pad of soft material;
   – retain the dressing and pad in position with a firm bandage;
   – see that the dressing and pad extend well above the level and beyond the edges of the wound.

If bleeding continues, apply further dressings and pads on top of the original dressing, and bandage more firmly.

6. Immobilise the injured part by a suitable method:—

— *for an upper limb* — a sling;

— *for a lower limb* — tying it to its fellow with adequate padding.

7. Remove carefully to hospital as soon as possible.

Treatment

Wounds from which foreign bodies cannot be removed: If it is not possible to remove the foreign body or if the ends of a broken bone protrude through the skin —

1. Apply pressure alongside the foreign body or broken bone, or press the sides of the wound firmly but gently together;

2. Apply a dressing over the wound;

Place pads of cotton wool or other soft material round the wound to a height sufficient to prevent pressure on the foreign body or projecting broken bone. A ring pad may be used. Secure with a bandage applied diagonally, thus avoiding the danger of pressure on the foreign body or broken bone.

Indirect pressure

If bleeding cannot be controlled by the application of direct pressure on the wound or when it is impossible to apply direct pressure successfully, it may be possible to apply indirect pressure at the appropriate pressure point between the heart and the wound. This pressure is not always successful owing to subsidiary bleeding.

A pressure point is where an important artery càn be compressed against an underlying bone to prevent the flow of blood beyond that point. Such pressure may be applied while dressing, pad and bandage are being prepared for application — not longer than 15 minutes.

Brachial pressure point

The brachial artery runs along the inner side of the muscles of each upper arm, its course being roughly indicated by the inner seam of a coat sleeve.

To apply pressure, pass your fingers under the casualty's upper arm and compress the artery against the bone (*humerus*) (Fig. 90).

Femoral pressure point

The femoral artery passes into each lower limb at a point corresponding to the centre of the fold of the groin.

Figure 90: Brachial
pressure point

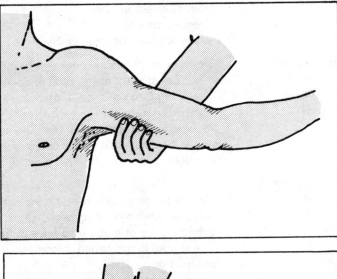

Figure 91: Femoral
pressure point

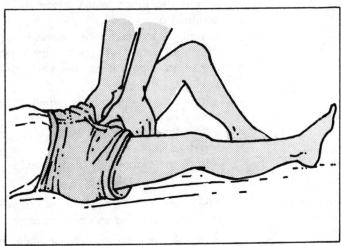

To apply pressure bend the casualty's knee, grasp his thigh with both hands and press directly and firmly downwards in the centre of the groin with both thumbs, one on top of the other against the brim of the pelvis (Fig. 91).

Internal bleeding

Internal bleeding may occur following an injury such as a broken bone, or result from a blow, or bullet; it may be associated with certain medical conditions in which there are no external causes.

Internal bleeding may —
— remain concealed;
— subsequently become visible.

Concealed

Bleeding may remain concealed in the following cases:—
— fracture of vault of the skull or cerebral bleeding;
— bleeding into the tissues, associated with fractures;
— bleeding from the spleen, liver or other organ into the abdomen. This source of bleeding is very dangerous and should be suspected when progressive signs and symptoms of bleeding develop following an injury to the abdomen.

Subsequently visible

Internal bleeding may become visible in the following ways:—
— when blood issues from the ear canal or nose or appears as a bloodshot eye, or is swallowed and afterwards vomited, as in the case of a fractured base of the skull;
— from the lungs when blood, bright red and frothy, is coughed up;
— from the stomach when blood is vomited. This blood will be bright red if vomited immediately, but will resemble coffee grounds if it has remained in the stomach for some time;
— from the upper bowel, when partly digested blood is passed in the motions, giving them a black tarry appearance;
— from the lower bowel, when blood, normal in appearance, is passed in the motions;
— from the kidneys or bladder, when blood escaping into the urine may make it smoky or red in appearance.

Treatment

The aim of First Aid is to obtain medical aid immediately and to combat shock.

1. Place the casualty at complete rest with legs raised; warn him not to move.
2. Loosen all tight clothing about his neck, chest and waist.
3. Reassure him and explain the necessity to relax mentally and physically.
4. Ensure that no other injuries are present; the casualty's word may be unreliable in severe cases.
5. Protect him from cold.
6. Remove him to hospital immediately in as quiet and gentle a manner as possible.
7. Keep careful watch on his breathing and pulse rate.

92

Make a written note of the pulse and time of recording for the Doctor. If removal to hospital is delayed, record pulse rate at 10–15 minute intervals. Keep record also of any specimens passed or vomited.

Do not give anything by the mouth.

Bleeding from special areas

From the scalp

Wounds of the scalp may cause severe and alarming bleeding.

Treatment

Do not press into or probe the wound – there may be an underlying fracture.
1. Apply a dressing much larger than the wound and bandage firmly in position.
2. If an underlying fracture is suspected or there is a foreign body in the wound, a large ring pad should be used to permit pressure around the wound, but not on the fracture or foreign body.
3. Refer casualty to doctor or to hospital for further treatment.

From the ear canal

Bleeding or perhaps the discharge of straw-coloured fluid from the ear canal may indicate a fracture of the base of the skull. (See page 111).

Treatment

1. Place a dressing or pad over the ear and secure lightly in position.
2. Lay the casualty carefully down with his head slightly raised and inclined to side of injury, or if unconscious, in the recovery position.
3. Remove to hospital immediately.
4. Keep careful watch on his breathing and pulse rate.

Do not pack the ear canal.

From the nose

Bleeding may be caused by a blow, but severe spontaneous bleeding, especially in the elderly, may be a sign of some medical condition, e.g. high blood pressure.
Bleeding is common from the area in the front part of the nose and due to a minor condition, e.g. when blowing or picking dry crusts, or when associated with hay fever or 'a cold'.

A fracture of the base of the skull may also cause blood to trickle from the nose (see page 111).

93

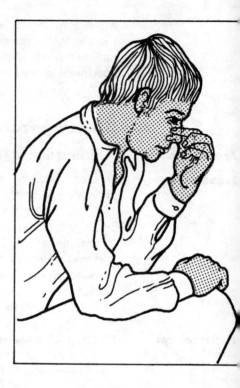

Figure 92: Treatment of nose bleed

Treatment

1. Support the casualty in a sitting position with his head slightly forward.
2. Instruct him to breathe through his mouth.
3. Tell him to pinch firmly the soft part of his nose for about ten minutes.
4. Loosen clothing about neck and chest.
5. Warn him not to blow his nose for some hours.
6. Do not disturb the clot.

If bleeding does not stop within a short time, or recurs, the casualty should receive medical attention.

From the gums

This occurs after extraction of teeth.

Treatment

1. Apply direct pressure by placing a gauze or cotton wool pad firmly on the socket. This pad must be large enough to prevent the teeth meeting when the pad is bitten on.
2. Instruct the casualty to bite on the pad for 10–20 minutes, supporting his chin with his hand. If bleeding is not controlled,

Figure 93: Treatment of bleeding from palm of the hand

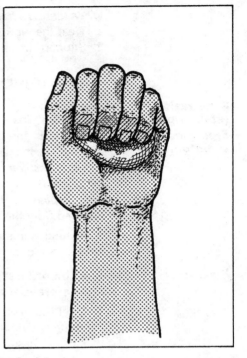

seek medical or dental advice.

Do not wash out the mouth, as this may disturb clotting.

Do not plug the socket.

From the tongue or cheek Compress the part between the finger and thumb, using a clean handkerchief or a dressing if available.

From the palm of the hand Bleeding may be severe as several blood vessels are involved.

Treatment
1. Apply direct pressure.
2. Raise the limb if possible.

When no fracture nor irremovable foreign body is present –
1. Cover the wound with a dressing;
2. Place a suitable pad over the dressing;
3. Bend the fingers over the pad so as to make a fist;
4. Bandage the fist firmly with a folded triangular bandage, tying off across the knuckles;
5. Support the limb in a triangular sling.

When there is a fracture or irremovable foreign body present —
1. Treat the wound;
2. Support the limb in a triangular sling.

Chest injuries

Penetrating (stab) wounds
Signs and symptoms

Blueness of lips and extremities may be present.
A wound in the chest wall may allow direct access of air into the chest cavity. If so —
— *during inspiration,* the noise of air being sucked in may be heard; (sucking wound) see page 122;
— *on expiration,* blood or blood-stained bubbles may be expelled from the wound.

If the lung is injured, the casualty may also cough up bright red frothy blood.

Treatment

The aim of First Aid is to seal the wound immediately and so prevent air entering the chest cavity.
1. Until the dressing can be applied, place the palm of the hand firmly over the wound.
2. Lay the casualty down with head and shoulders raised and the body inclined towards the injured side.
3. Plug the wound lightly with a dressing.
4. Cover the dressing with a thick layer of cotton wool.
5. Retain it firmly in position by strapping or a bandage.
6. **Remove urgently to hospital.**

Stove-in chest

An increasingly common example is the 'steering wheel injury', caused when the driver of a motor vehicle is flung violently forward against the steering wheel. There may be a fracture of several ribs and of the breast-bone, parts of which may be driven inwards possibly damaging the heart, lungs, liver or spleen, with the danger of internal bleeding.
A severe compression injury may also cause this condition.

Signs and symptoms

The casualty is severely distressed with difficult breathing.
Blueness of his lips and extremities may be present.
The injured part of the chest wall will be seen to have lost its rigidity. Instead of moving normally with the remainder of the chest, it does the opposite — during inspiration it is sucked in; on expiration it is blown out.

Sufficient air does not enter the lungs and in consequence the blood cannot obtain enough oxygen.

Treatment

The aim of First Aid is to reduce respiratory activity to the minimum necessary.

1. Loosen any tight clothing — collar, belt etc.
2. Place the casualty at rest, raise head of stretcher to reduce pressure of abdominal contents on diaphragm.
3. Immobilise the injured part of the chest wall by placing the arm with the elbow bent against it as a splint.
4. Secure by strapping or bandaging the arm to the chest.
5. **Remove urgently to hospital.**

Blast injuries

Caused by an explosion.

Signs and symptoms

The casualty may be apprehensive and in a tremulous state;
Pain in the chest with restlessness;
Blueness of lips and extremities may be present;
Frothy blood-stained sputum may be coughed up;
Breathing may be difficult.

There may be no signs of bruising or of fractures.

On examination, the casualty may not complain of pain or tenderness.

Treatment

1. Reassure him, insisting that complete rest is essential.
2. Loosen any tight clothing — collar, belt, etc.
3. Lay him down with head and shoulders raised and supported (*semi-recumbent position*).
4. **Remove urgently to hospital.**

Wounds of the abdominal wall

Treatment

Place the casualty so that the wound does not gape — generally on his back with head and shoulders slightly raised and supported, with a pillow under his knees.

If no internal organs protrude —
— apply a dressing to the wound and bandage firmly in position.

If internal organs protrude through the wound —
— cover lightly with a soft clean towel or a large gauze dressing;

97

– secure without undue pressure.

Do not attempt to replace protruding organs.

In all cases –
– support the abdomen if vomiting or coughing is present.
– **remove urgently to hospital.**

Do not give anything by mouth.

Crush injuries

This is a condition in which it is of great importance to prevent acute kidney failure, which is liable to occur if casualties have been crushed or trapped for more than an hour by some heavy weight, such as fallen masonry or machinery.

Crush injury involves soft tissues (muscle and skin) and sometimes bones are fractured.

On release, such casualties may show little sign of injury except perhaps redness or swelling of the part. There may be some bruising or blister formation and casualties may complain of numbness and tingling.

Complications may occur some hours after release when the injured tissues may swell and become hard due to the out-pouring of fluid (plasma) from the blood into them. Blood pressure falls and shock becomes profound. Certain poisonous products of the injured muscles are absorbed into the blood stream and can lead to acute kidney failure and death.

Treatment

The aim of First Aid is to prevent a dangerous fall in the blood pressure and failure of the kidneys.

1. On release, keep the casualty on his back with head low and lower limbs raised if possible. Warn him not to move.

2. Arrange for removal to hospital with least delay, as this is the danger period. It is important to inform the hospital of the possibility of crush injury as initially there may be little evidence to suggest it.

3. If he is conscious and an internal abdominal injury is not suspected give an adult casualty sips of iced water to wash out his mouth, otherwise no other fluid is to be offered as he may require an anaesthetic on admission to hospital.

Figures 94 and 95: Treatment of bleeding from varicose veins

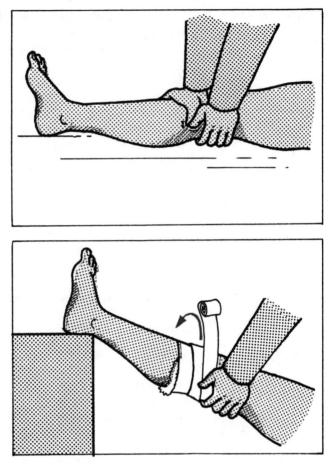

4. Reassure the casualty.
5. Leave an injured limb uncovered.

Varicose veins

Varicose veins occur when the valves in the veins, usually those of the legs, fail to act properly. There is back pressure and the veins enlarge, forming a reservoir of blood.

Bleeding from a burst varicose vein in the leg may be *sudden and severe,* and if not immediately controlled may quickly be fatal.

Treatment	1. Apply immediate direct pressure with the hand to the bleeding point. 2. Loosen any constriction, such as garter, which may impede the circulation. 3. Lay casualty flat on his back and raise the leg as high as possible. 4. Apply a dressing, pad and bandage firmly in position. 5. Keep the leg raised and supported. 6. Ensure that the casualty is seen by his own doctor or taken to hospital.

Bruise (contusion)

A bruise is bleeding beneath the unbroken skin often due to a fall or a blow on the surface of the body. It is a minor form of internal bleeding, but could be severe if the area involved is extensive.

The injury is usually accompanied by pain, discoloration and swelling.

Before treatment check there are no further injuries present.

Treatment	1. Put the part at rest in the most comfortable position. 2. Apply a cold application to reduce swelling and to relieve pain. Cold applications include – – cold compress; – ice bag.
Cold compress	Soak a thin towel, large handkerchief, piece of flannel or absorbent cotton wool in cold water. Squeeze out the surplus water and apply the compress to the bruised area. Keep it cool by dripping water on it as required, or replace it by further compresses. Ensure good evaporation by not covering the compress, but, if necessary, use open weave material to keep it in place.
Ice bag	Fill a polythene (or non-porous) bag two-thirds full with crushed ice. Add some common salt to melt the ice and increase the cooling action. Expel the air and tie up the bag. Wrap the bag in a thin towel and apply it carefully to the bruised part. Renew ice and salt as necessary.

Acute heart attacks

These result from a reduction in the blood supply to the muscular wall of the heart.

There are two varieties –
– angina pectoris (severe pain in the chest);
– obstruction of a coronary artery in the wall of the heart.

Angina pectoris

The channels of the arteries supplying blood to the heart have become too narrow for an adequate supply to the heart muscle, when it is working harder than normal. Excitement or over-exertion brings on an attack of pain in the chest, which often spreads to the left shoulder and arm and to the fingers. The pain may also spread to the throat and jaws and to the other upper limb. It is relieved by rest and usually lasts only a few minutes.

Coronary obstruction

The blood clots suddenly in a coronary artery and blocks it. The onset of pain is not necessarily related to exertion. The casualty is gripped by an excruciating vice-like pain behind the breast-bone; it may radiate into the upper limbs, throat or jaw. Rest is essential, but may not ease the pain.

Signs and symptoms

In both varieties the casualty suffers severely from shock and –
– severe pain may force him to stop what he is doing and sit down or lean against a wall for support;
– he may feel giddy and sink to the ground. Even when

Figure 96:
The semi-recumbent
position

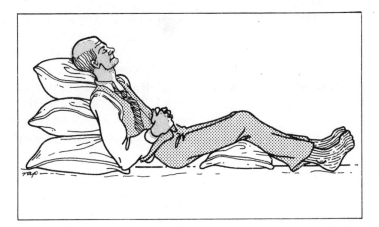

shock is slight the casualty may still be seriously ill as a further severe attack may follow;
— he is often short of breath;
— he may become unconscious;
— the pulse is weak and may be irregular.

Note: In coronary obstruction death may result from the stopping of the heart beat.

Treatment

The aim of First Aid is to reduce the work of the heart and sustain the casualty during an attack.

1. *Do not* move the casualty unnecessarily but place him in the most comfortable position, which is usually —
— semi-recumbent with his head and shoulders raised on two or more pillows; *or*
— supported in a sitting position if this makes his breathing easier.

2. Loosen clothing about neck, chest and waist.

3. If breathing fails, begin artificial respiration immediately, and if necessary give external heart compression. Both these procedures may have to be continued on the way to hospital.

4. Arrange for urgent transport to hospital, obtaining medical aid if available. Administration of oxygen may be required.

Note: People liable to heart pain (*angina*) often carry tablets (glyceril trinitrate) which are useful for the prevention of an attack but not in treatment.

Congestive heart failure

During chronic heart disease, heart failure and collapse may occur. The condition is different from coronary obstruction. It resembles that of an acute heart attack, but the casualty may be cyanosed and may cough up large amounts of blood-stained sputum.

Treatment

As for Acute Heart Attack, but support the casualty in a sitting position. *Do not lay* him flat as he will not be able to get sufficient air into his lungs and may become asphyxiated.

Be prepared to deal with vomiting and bowel action.

CHAPTER SEVEN

Shock

Shock is a condition resulting from a lessening of the activities of the vital functions of the body arising from a lack of blood supply. It may accompany injuries, severe pain or sudden illness. The severity of shock depends upon the nature and extent of the injury or other cause and may vary from a feeling of faintness even to death, and is associated with many conditions and injuries.

Causes

Severe bleeding
External – for example, from an artery or ruptured varicose vein.
Internal – for example, into the abdomen, the chest cavity or the tissues surrounding the broken bone of a limb.

Loss of plasma from the circulation
Burns; crush injuries.

Heart failure
Acute heart attacks.

Acute abdominal emergencies
Perforation of the stomach, ruptured appendix.

Loss of body fluid
Recurrent vomiting (sea-sickness, intestinal obstruction) or severe diarrhoea (acute gastroenteritis, dysentery, cholera).

Nerve stimulation
Nerve shock is caused by sensory nerve stimulation, usually, but not always, painful.

Signs and symptoms

Casualty will become extremely pale;
– his skin cold and clammy with profuse sweating;
– he may feel faint or giddy or have blurring of vision;
– he may feel sick and may vomit;
– he may complain of thirst;
– he may be very anxious;
– consciousness may be clouded;

103

– his pulse increases in rate; tending to become weak and thready;

– his breathing is shallow and rapid.

Treatment

1. Lay casualty down and deal with the injury or underlying cause of the shock.

2. Waste no time – get the casualty to hospital – his life may depend upon immediate blood transfusion and other hospital treatment.

3. Keep his head low and turned to one side with the lower limbs raised when possible;

or if there is an injury to his head, chest or abdomen, the shoulders should be raised slightly and supported, with his head turned to one side;

or if vomiting seems likely or if he is unconscious, place him carefully in the recovery position.

4. Loosen clothing at the neck, chest and waist.

5. If the casualty complains of thirst, moisten his lips with water.

6. Protect him when necessary with a blanket or sheet.

7. Keep frequent records of the pulse and respiration rates if removal to hospital is likely to be delayed.

Do not heat the casualty or use hot water bottles, as this draws blood from the vital organs to the skin.

Do not give the casualty anything to drink.

Do not move him unnecessarily. Leaving the casualty in the position found frequently outweighs the benefits of any other action. The more serious the injury, the more important it is *not* to move the casualty more than is necessary.

Fainting

Fainting follows a temporary inadequate supply of blood to the brain, frequently caused by some emotional or sensory stimulus. It may begin with a feeling of faintness, or there may be a sudden collapse. Some degree of nerve shock accompanies all injuries.

Causes

A fright, bad news, a horrifying sight or pain.

Fatigue or long periods of sitting or standing in a hot stuffy atmosphere.

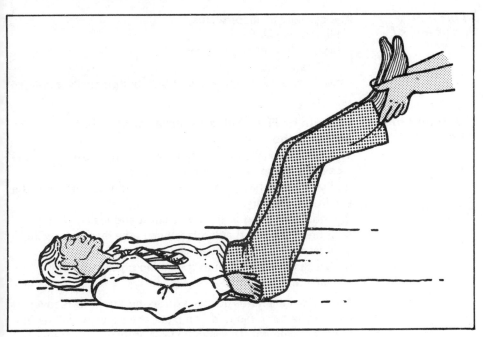

Figure 97: Treatment of a faint.

Debilitating illness.
Injury to some part of the body.

Impending faint

There may be some warning before fainting – the person may yawn or sway and feel unsteady and become giddy; his face becomes pale or greenish white in colour, and beads of sweat are seen on his face, neck and hands; his consciousness clouds.

Treatment of impending faint

1. Reassure him and urge him to breathe deeply, to flex the muscles of his legs, thighs and buttocks and so help the circulation of the blood.
2. Loosen clothing at the neck, chest and waist.
3. Lay him down in a current of fresh air until his colour returns, or it may be more convenient to sit him down and lower his head between his knees.
4. On recovery, sips of water may be given.
5. Smelling salts may be useful. Test strength before use.

Signs and symptoms of a faint

The casualty is unconscious;
– his face is pale;
– his skin is cold and clammy;
– his breathing is shallow;
– his pulse is weak and slow at first, but gradually increases in rate.

Treatment of a faint

The aim of First Aid is to get a satisfactory supply of blood to the brain.
1. Lay the casualty down and deal with any cause. Raise the legs slightly above the level of his head.
2. See that he has plenty of fresh air and put him into the shade, if necessary.
3. Loosen clothing at the neck, chest and waist.
4. If breathing is difficult, place him in the recovery position.
5. Reassure him as he regains consciousness.
6. Gradually raise him into the sitting position and give sips of water, if requested.

Note: Colour returns to his skin as he starts to recover. If recovery is not rapid and complete, the casualty will require hospital treatment. This is more likely if there is an associated injury.

CHAPTER EIGHT

Injuries to bones

Fractures

A fracture is a broken or cracked bone.

In young children, the break may be incomplete and is referred to as a greenstick fracture.

Where the diagnosis is uncertain, all doubtful cases should be considered as fractures.

Causes of fractures

Direct force – when the bone breaks at the spot where the force is applied, e.g. from a kick or blow.

Indirect force – (*a*) when the bone breaks at some distance from the spot where the force is applied. In such cases the force is transmitted along the intervening bones which usually escape injury, e.g. fracture of the collar-bone may result from a fall on the outstretched hand.
(*b*) when there is a sudden violent contraction of muscles which may cause a fracture, e.g., of the knee-cap or the tip of the elbow.

Types of fractures

Closed – where the skin surface is not broken.

Open – when there is a wound leading down to the fracture, or when the fractured ends protrude through the skin, thus allowing germs to gain access to soft tissues and broken bone.

When there is associated injury to an important structure such as the brain, major blood vessels, nerves, lungs, liver, or when associated with a dislocation of a joint, either type of fracture is said to be 'complicated'.

Signs and symptoms

Pain – at or near the site of the fracture. Made worse by movement of the injured part.

Tenderness – on gentle pressure over the affected part.

107

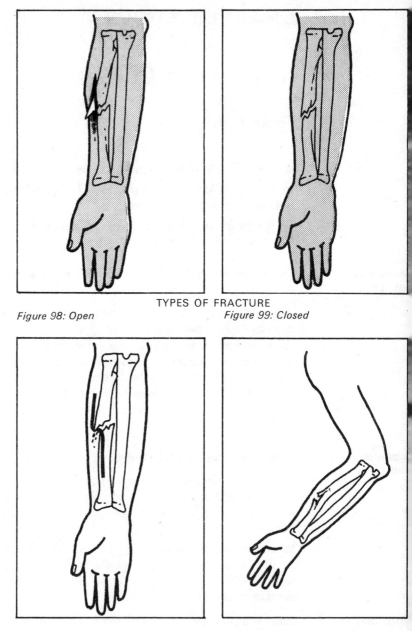

TYPES OF FRACTURE

Figure 98: Open *Figure 99: Closed*

Figure 100: An example of a complicated fracture

Figure 101: An example of a greenstick fracture

Swelling – the result of blood loss into the tissues, may later be accompanied by bruising. Swelling may prevent the recognition of other signs, so when in doubt treat as a fracture.

Loss of control – the casualty is unable to move the injured part normally.

Deformity – such as –
– *irregularity of the bone* – if the fracture is near the skin, the irregularity may be seen or felt;
– *shortening of the limb* – due to contraction of the muscles causing the broken ends of the bone to override each other;
– *angulation or rotation of a limb* – due to a fracture of some supporting bone, e.g. the neck of the femur – the foot falls outwards;
– *depression of a flat bone* – as in the skull.

Unnatural movement – at the seat of the fracture, unless the broken ends are driven into each other.

A coarse bony grating (crepitus) – may be felt or heard during the examination of an injured part if the ends of a broken bone move against each other, but this should never deliberately be sought.

Shock – increased by the loss of blood from the circulation. In addition to the above, the snap of the bone may have been felt or heard. It must also be clearly understood that all the above signs and symptoms may not be present in every fracture. As many signs as possible should be noted by simple observation and without moving any part unnecessarily, as this may cause pain or further damage.

Compare the injured and uninjured limbs whenever possible.

General rules for treatment

1. Asphyxia, bleeding and severe wounds must be dealt with before dealing with any fracture.
2. Treat the fracture on the site of the incident, unless life is endangered (the casualty's or your own), in which case temporary fixation should be carried out before moving the casualty as short a distance as possible.
3. Steady and, if necessary, support the injured part at once to prevent further damage, and maintain this control until the fracture has been immobilised.

4. Immobilise by using –

– *body bandages* – using the casualty's body as a means of support will prove adequate for normal purposes.

– *splints and bandages* – the support of splints may be required when there is a possibility of a long or rough journey before medical aid is available, or in the presence of multiple injuries.

5. Raise the injured part after immobilisation if possible, in order to reduce discomfort and swelling.

Use of bandages for fractures

Bandages should be applied sufficiently firmly to prevent movement but not so tightly as to interfere with the circulation of the blood or to cause pain.

Separate skin surfaces with soft padding before bandaging together, in order to prevent discomfort and chafing of the skin.

Always tie knots over a splint or on the uninjured side. If both lower limbs are injured, tie the knots in front between them.

Check at 15 minute intervals to ensure that they are not becoming too tight as a result of swelling of the injured tissues. This is especially important when an elbow has been injured and is supported in a sling.

To pass bandages underneath him if the casualty is lying down, use the natural hollows of the body, e.g. the neck, loins, knees.

Use of splints

If splints are required, they should be –
– sufficiently rigid;
– long enough to immobilise the joint above and below the fracture;
– well padded and wide enough to fit comfortably to the limb;
– applied over clothing.

In emergencies, a splint may be improvised from a walking stick, umbrella, broom handle, piece of wood, cardboard or firmly folded newspaper or magazine.

Disposal

All casualties who have fractures or suspected fractures must be sent to hospital for further attention.

Transport of the casualty should be as gentle as possible.

Special fractures

The skull

The fracture is often complicated by some injury to the brain and may produce varying degrees of unconsciousness (see 'Unconsciousness', page 140).

Fracture of the vault (cranium): This is caused by a direct blow or fall on the upper part or sides of the skull; part of the bone may be depressed inwards.

Fracture of the base: This is usually the result of indirect force — a severe blow to the lower jaw or a fall on to the feet or lower part of the spine, transmitting the force to the base of the skull.

Signs and symptoms

Blood or straw-coloured fluid may sometimes issue from the ear canal or from the nose; or it may be swallowed and afterwards vomited. The fracture may involve the orbit causing a bloodshot eye and later a 'black eye'.

Treatment

1. Place the casualty in the recovery position with adequate support.
2. Establish as soon as possible, level of consciousness and check frequently.
3. If blood or fluid comes from the ear canal, apply a sterile dressing and secure lightly in place.
4. Keep a careful check on the casualty's breathing — ensure a clear airway; start artificial respiration if breathing begins to fail or stops.
5. Maintain the casualty's position during transport and avoid all unnecessary movement.

Jaw and face injuries

Fractures and wounds may be complicated by damage to the brain. The skull or cervical spine may also be injured.

The following serious risks are associated with these injuries:—
Obstruction of the casualty's airway with resulting asphyxia by —
— the tongue falling to the back of the throat of an unconscious casualty;
— swelling of tissues following the injury;
— displaced and lacerated tissues.

Inadequate or absent cough reflex — which allows secretions,

111

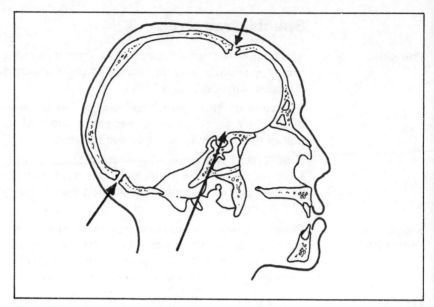

Figure 102: Fracture sites of the skull

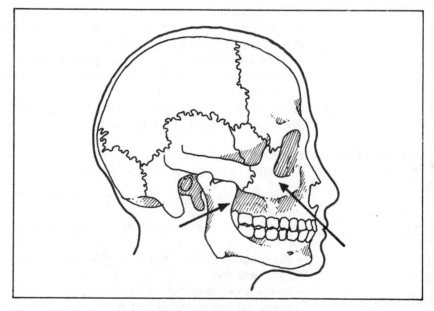

Figure 103: Common fracture sites of the face and jaw

blood and foreign material to drain unnoticed into the lungs, causing infection and complications such as collapse of the lungs;

bleeding – which initially may be profuse and alarming, but which is not usually prolonged and should be controlled by direct pressure.

Fracture of lower jaw

This is always the result of direct force, for example, a severe blow to the jaw, and there is usually a wound inside the mouth. Usually, only one side of the jaw is affected.

Signs and symptoms

Pain increased by jaw movements or by swallowing;
Difficulty in speaking;
Excessive flow of saliva, which is frequently blood-stained;
Irregularity of the teeth;
Swelling, tenderness and, later, bruising of the face and lower jaw.
Severe bleeding if tongue is injured.

Treatment

The primary aim of First Aid in jaw and face injuries is to maintain respiration.
1. Maintain an open airway – ensure tongue has not fallen to the back of the throat and that the mouth is not obstructed.
2. Control bleeding.
3. Remove any false or detached teeth.
4. Support the jaw with a soft pad held in place by hand or by a suitable bandage.
5. **The conscious casualty –**
not severely injured may sit up with his head well forward so that any secretions can drain freely;
severely injured, with downward displacement of the chin and associated soft tissues, may require to be kept in the recovery position.

The unconscious casualty –
– must be placed in the recovery position, making sure that the jaw is kept well forward.
6. If the casualty seems likely to vomit, turn his head to the sound side, supporting the jaw with the palm of your hand.
7. **Arrange for urgent removal to hospital.**

Fracture of spine

This is a grave and serious injury. If the casualty is not correctly handled, the spinal cord may be permanently

113

Figure 104: Fracture of the spine (cervical)

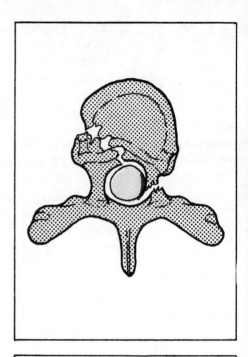

Figure 105: Fracture of the spine (lumbar)

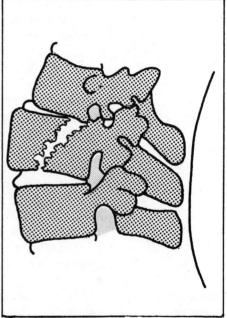

damaged and paralysis result.

Causes of fractures

Direct force such as —
– a fall of a heavy weight across the casualty's back;
– a fall from a height on to the back across a bar;
– impact in a vehicle collision.

Indirect force such as —
– a heavy fall on the feet or buttocks;
– a fall on the head from a height as in diving;
– over-flexion or jerking of the spine as in a vehicle collision.

The fracture may be complicated by injury to the spinal cord or to the nerves issuing from it, causing complete or partial loss of power (paralysis) and/or sensation in all parts of the body below the site of the injury.

Fracture of the spine should always be suspected in all cases in which there is a history of accident or injury to the vertebral column and the casualty complains of pain in his back.

All such cases must be regarded as serious emergencies and any doubtful case treated as a fracture.

Signs and symptoms

Casualty is found collapsed and complains of severe pain in his back.

He sometimes states that he feels cut in half, that his lower limbs are numb, or that he has lost control of them.

Possible loss of power in the limbs; ask the casualty to —
– move his wrists and ankles;
– move his fingers and toes.

Possible loss of sensation; test by gently touching the limbs without his knowledge and asking casualty if he can feel touch or pain.

Even though there is no apparent loss of power or sensation, handle with the utmost care and so prevent a spinal fracture from causing damage to the spinal cord.

Treatment

The aim of First Aid is to prepare the casualty so that he can be moved and transported to the hospital without damaging the spinal cord.

1. Warn the casualty to lie still.

2. **If medical aid is readily available —**
– *do not* move the casualty;

– cover him with a blanket and await the arrival of the doctor.

If medical aid is not readily available –

– whilst the casualty's shoulders and pelvis are firmly held, place pads of soft material between the thighs, knees and ankles;

– tie the ankles and feet together with a figure-of-eight bandage;

– apply broad bandages round –

(*i*) the thighs;

(*ii*) the knees.

Position of casualty

The conscious casualty is best transported in the face-upwards position, and this is essential in suspected fractures of the neck.

The unconscious casualty should be carefully supported with rolled blankets, pillows, etc., in the face-upwards position. The recovery position must not be used because of risk of further damage to the spinal cord. (This is the only exception to this general rule governing the recovery position). The breathing must be carefully and continuously watched and if it ceases, an airway must be achieved even by tilting the head backwards preparatory to mouth-to-mouth resuscitation if this becomes necessary.

Note: This is an example of the calculated risk since injury may result but otherwise death is certain. (See page 174)

Preparation of stretcher

The canvas bed of a stretcher should be stiffened by placing short boards across it. If these are not available a narrow shutter, a door or board at least as wide and as long as the casualty may be used.

Cover the boards with a folded blanket, then 'blanket the stretcher' (see page 184).

Accurately place pads on the stretcher to support the natural curves of the casualty's neck, small of back, knees and ankles.

Placing a blanket under casualty

When the casualty is not already lying on a blanket or rug and one is available –

1. Roll the blanket or rug lengthwise for half its width; place the roll in line with and against the casualty;

2. While two First Aiders maintain firm control of the head and lower limbs, the other First Aiders slowly and gently turn the casualty as in one piece on to his side, without bending the neck or twisting the trunk. The two First Aiders controlling the head and the lower limbs must maintain an even tension while the casualty is being turned.

3. The rolled portion of the blanket or rug is then moved up to the casualty's back.

4. The casualty is then gently turned back over the roll of the blanket or rug on to his opposite side.

5. The blanket or rug is then unrolled and the casualty gently turned on to his back.

Blanket Lift

Loading the stretcher

1. Roll the two edges of the blanket up against the sides of the casualty. If poles of sufficient length and rigidity are available the edges of the blanket should be rolled round them. This will make the lifting of the casualty much easier and prevent sagging;

2. While the two First Aiders continue to support the head and the lower limbs, the remaining First Aiders place themselves on each side of the casualty, facing one another;

3. The First Aiders acting together, grasp the rolled edges of the blanket, carefully and evenly lift the casualty to a sufficient height to enable the stretcher to be pushed underneath. It will be necessary for the First Aider supporting the feet to keep his legs apart to allow the stretcher to be pushed between them.

If it is not possible to push the stretcher under the casualty, it should be placed close to the casualty's head or feet, and after carefully lifting the casualty the First Aiders should move with short even side paces until the casualty is directly over the stretcher.

Before lowering him on the stretcher, ensure that the pads are in the correct position. With neck injuries place firm supports at each side of the head to steady it.

Lifting with slings

In special circumstances slings may be made from broad bandages, roller towels, webbing bands (C.D. pattern) etc., and passed under the casualty's neck, shoulders, small of

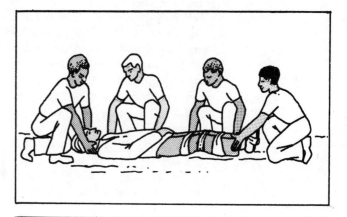

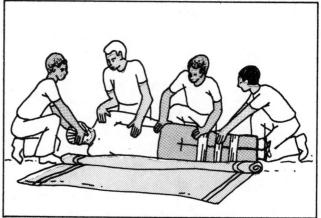

Figure 108: Blanket lift:
Lifting

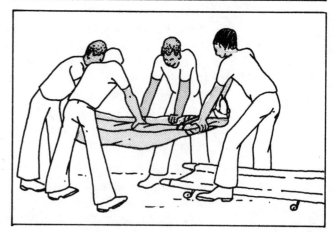

Figures 109, 110 and 111:
Lifting with webbing bands

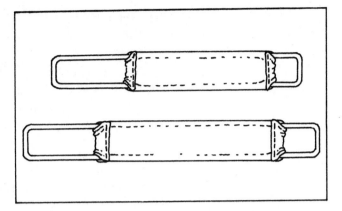

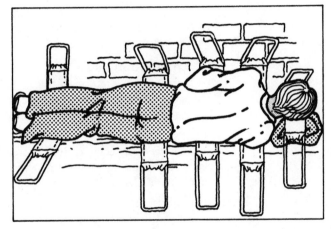

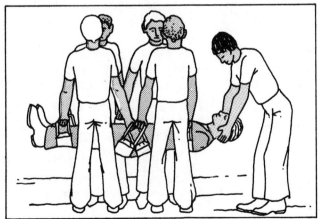

back, knees and ankles.

The ends of the slings are tied to stout poles, one on each side of the casualty.

Test that when the weight is taken up, there will be an even tension of all slings.

With one First Aider supporting his head, the casualty is then loaded on to a stretcher in the same way as for a blanket lift.

Lifting with webbing bands (Civil Defence)

These bands, if available, can facilitate the moving and lifting of a casualty. They are made in two lengths —

— *those of 2 ft.* are used for lifting at the head, neck or feet;
— *those of 3 ft.* are used for lifting under the chest, small of back and the hips.

The **method of use** is —

— grasping the junction of the webbing and the long handle, slide the handle under the casualty; the band can then be gently drawn through until there is a handle on each side of him.

— if the casualty is lying close to the wall and it is not possible without disturbing him to pass the long handle through, the short handle is tied to or bent over the long handle and then slid under the casualty.

— when the bands are applied and the casualty's head and the lower limbs are steadied, he can be raised and lifted on to a stretcher.

Removal to hospital

It is important that spinal injuries be transported in as gentle a way as possible. More harm is likely to result from a fast rough ride than from a slow smooth one.

He may be lifted on to the stretcher in the position in which he is found, unless his neck is injured when he must be placed face upwards.

If transported on his side, steady the casualty with rolled blankets, pillows etc.

Retain in position by bandaging over the casualty and under the stretcher.

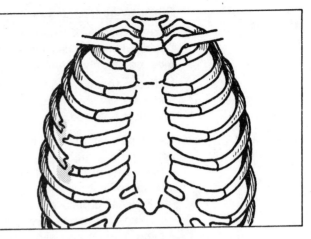

Figure 112: Fracture of the ribs

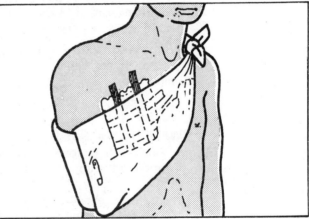

Figure 113: Fracture of the ribs (complicated): first stage of treatment

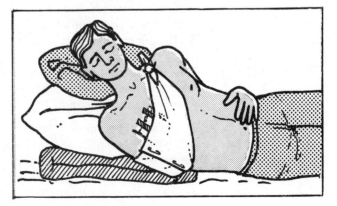

Figure 114: Fracture of the ribs (complicated): second stage of treatment

Fracture of the ribs

Ribs may be fractured by –

Direct force – if severe; the broken ends of the bone may be driven inwards causing a complicated fracture. The organs most commonly involved are the lungs.

Indirect force – usually produced by pressure on the front and back of the chest, as in crushing. Usually more than one rib is involved.

Signs and symptoms

Sharp pain at the site of the fracture, increased by deep breathing or coughing;
– the casualty usually takes short, shallow breaths in an attempt to limit movement and decrease pain;
– if internal organs are affected, there may be signs and symptoms of internal bleeding;
– there may be an open wound in the chest wall over the fracture, causing a 'sucking wound' of the chest which will lead to asphyxia unless treated immediately.

Treatment

When the fracture is uncomplicated:
1. Support the upper limb on the injured side in an arm sling.

2. Transport as a sitting or walking case unless otherwise indicated.

When the fracture is complicated:
1. Any 'sucking wound' must be made airtight immediately.
2. Support the upper limb on the injured side in a triangular sling.
3. Lay the casualty down with head and shoulders raised, and the body inclined towards the injured side.
4. Support the casualty in this position by means of a folded blanket applied lengthwise to his back.
5. Transport to hospital as a stretcher case.

The breastbone

This fracture is usually associated with crush injuries and may be complicated by damage to the underlying chest organs and blood vessels.

Treatment

1. Loosen tight clothing about neck, chest and waist.
2. Place the casualty with his head and shoulders raised in the most comfortable position, with due regard to associated injuries.
3. Transport as stretcher case.

Collar-bone
Causes

Indirect force – the usual cause – a fall on the outstretched hand or on the point of the shoulder.

Direct force – by a blow.

Signs and symptoms

Pain and tenderness at the site of the injury;
– the arm on the injured side is partly helpless;
– the casualty supports it at the elbow and keeps his head inclined towards the injured side. This relieves his pain by reducing muscle tension;
– swelling or deformity can be seen or felt over the site of the fracture.

Treatment

1. Fold two triangular bandages narrow.
2. Pass each narrow bandage through one arm pit, encircle the same shoulder and tie behind in a reef knot.
3. Carry the free ends across the back over a pad placed between the shoulder blades; tie opposite ends together, or secure with a third bandage.
As the knots are carefully tightened the shoulders are braced well back, in order to correct the overriding of the broken ends of the clavicle.
4. Support the arm on the injured side in a triangular arm sling.

Shoulder-blade

This rare injury is the result of direct force.

Treatment

1. Remove overcoat and braces.
2. Place a pad in the armpit.
3. Support the upper limb in a triangular sling, with finger-tips to opposite shoulder.
4. Give further support by securing the upper limb to the chest by a broad bandage applied over the sling.

The upper limb

Upper arm: May occur anywhere along the bone (humerus) and be near or even involve the elbow joint.
Forearm: May involve either the radius or ulna or both bones and also the elbow joint.

Treatment

If elbow is not involved:
1. Place the forearm across the chest, finger tips touching the fold of the opposite armpit.
2. Ensure adequate soft padding between the limb and the chest.
3. Support the limb in an arm sling.

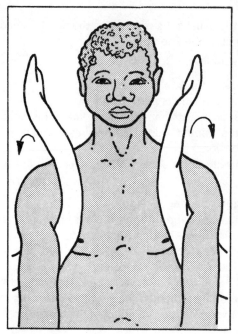

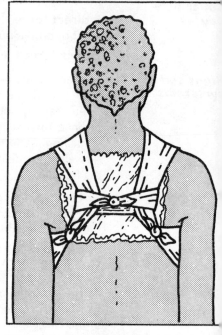

Figures 115, 116 and 117:
Treatment of a fractured
clavicle, stages 1, 2 and 3

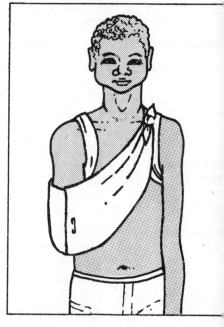

124

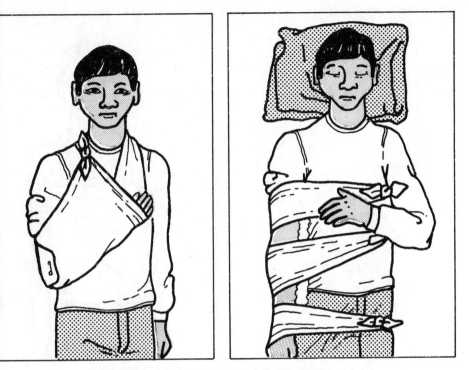

Figures 118 and 119: Treatment of fracture of the humerus

4. Give further support by securing the upper limb to the chest by a broad bandage applied over the sling.

If elbow cannot be flexed:

1. *Do not* attempt to force it.

2. Lay casualty down.

3. Place the limb gently by the casualty's side, palm to thigh.

4. Protect with adequate soft padding between the limb and the body.

5. Secure by three broad bandages, tied on the uninjured side of the body —
(*i*)   round upper arm and trunk;
(*ii*) round forearm and trunk;
(*iii*) round the wrist and thighs.

6. Transport as a stretcher case.

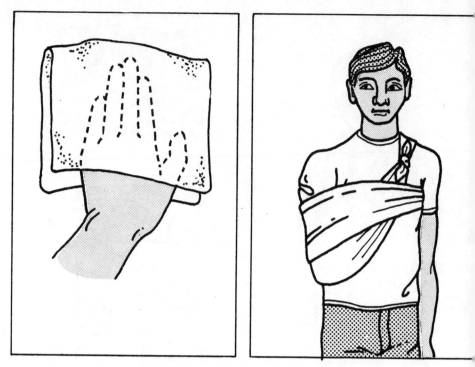

Figures 120 and 121: Treatment of a fractured finger

Wrist and lower end of forearm – when the lower end of the radius is fractured (Colles's fracture) there may or may not be considerable deformity present. It is a common fracture and can be mistaken for a sprain of the wrist.

Treatment

1. Protect the forearm and wrist by placing it on a fold of soft padding.
2. Support the limb in an arm sling.
3. Give further support by securing the upper limb to the chest by a broad bandage applied over the sling.

Hands and fingers – fractures may be complicated by severe bleeding into the tissues.

Treatment

1. Protect the hand by placing it on a fold of soft material.
2. Support the limb in a triangular sling.
3. Give further support by securing the upper limb to the chest by a broad bandage applied over the sling.

126

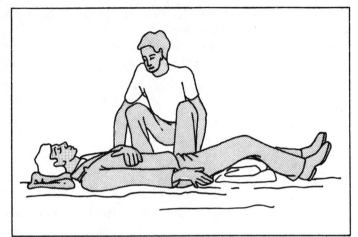

Figure: 122 Fracture of the pelvis

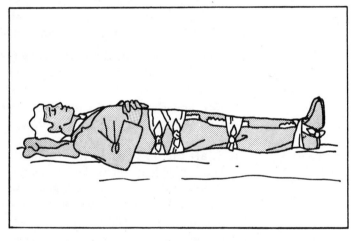

Figure 123: Preparation for a long or rough journey

The pelvis	This may be complicated by injury to organs of the pelvis, especially the bladder and urinary passages, and by internal bleeding.
Causes	**Direct force** – as by a heavy fall of debris, or being knocked down by a motor vehicle.
	Indirect force – falling from a height and landing heavily on both feet when lower limbs are held stiffly.
Signs and symptoms	Pain in the region of the hips and loins, increased by movement;

127

— inability to stand, despite the absence of injury to the lower limbs;

— there may be a desire to pass water frequently, though with difficulty. If passed, the urine may be darkened by blood.

Treatment

1. Lay the casualty down in the most comfortable position — usually on his back with knees straight.

If he wishes to bend knees slightly, they should be supported on a folded blanket.

2. Tell him not to pass water on any account.

3. **If journey to hospital is short and smooth —**
— transport as a stretcher case in the same position.

If journey to hospital is likely to be rough or there may be some delay in reaching hospital —

(*i*) Apply two broad bandages round the pelvis, overlapping by half, and their centres in line with the hip joints of the affected side. Tie off on the uninjured side.

The bandages should be sufficiently firm to support the part.

(*ii*) Place adequate soft padding between the knees and the ankles.

(*iii*) Apply a figure-of-eight bandage round the ankles and feet, and a broad bandage round the knees.

Lower limb

Shaft of the thigh bone (femur)
The femur may be broken anywhere along its length. In infants and in the aged, a fracture may result from a minor injury, otherwise considerable violence is required.

Fractures of the femur must always be regarded as serious injuries because of the great shock accompanied by loss of blood into the surrounding tissues.

Neck of the thigh bone (femur)
This occurs usually in elderly people, often through a relatively slight cause such as tripping. It may be mistaken for a badly bruised hip.

An elderly person who, after a fall or minor injury, complains of pain in the region of the hip with some disability, should be considered to have a fracture of the neck of the femur, until some other diagnosis in hospital has been established. In women, a skirt may be used as padding between the limbs.

Figure 124: Fracture of
neck of femur and of
shaft

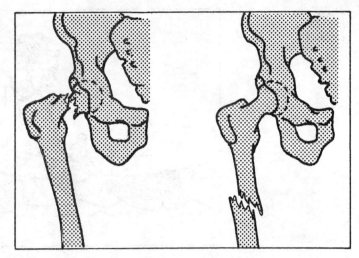

Figure 125: Typical
position – foot fallen
outwards

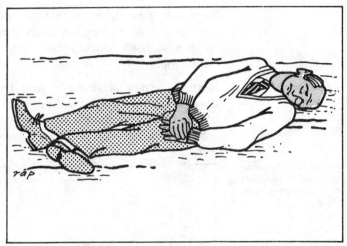

The Leg

One or both bones may be broken. Commonly a fracture of
the tibia is open.

A fracture of the fibula two or three inches above the ankle
(Pott's fracture) may be mistaken for a sprain of the ankle
joint.

Fractures of the major bones of the lower limb

Treatment

1. Steady and support the injured limb.
2. Bring the sound limb gently to the side of the injured one.

129

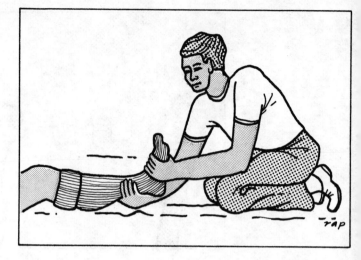

Figure 126: Treatment of fracture of tibia or fibula

3. Should it be necessary to move the injured limb, gentle traction should be applied and maintained until the two limbs have been tied together. This may cause temporary discomfort.

Transport

If the journey is smooth, and the casualty can be comfortably removed to hospital within half an hour of the arrival of the ambulance –
– place adequate soft padding between the thighs, knees

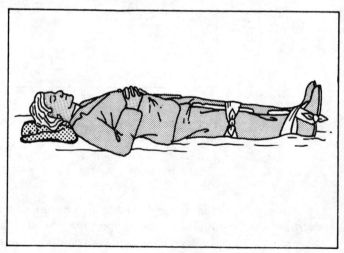

Figure 127: Treatment of casualty with fracture of lower limb: smooth journey

and ankles.

– secure by tying together with two broad bandages –

(*i*)   the ankles and feet with a figure-of-eight bandage;

(*ii*)   the knees.

If journey is likely to be rough or long

When no splints are available further secure by three broad bandages –

(*iii*)   the legs;

(*iv*)   the thighs;

(*v*)   below site of fracture ('floater' bandage).

When splints are available

(*a*)   **For a fractured leg –**

(*i*)   apply well-padded splint between the limbs, extending from the crutch to the foot;

(*ii*)   immobilise with five bandages as described above.

(*b*)   **For a fractured thigh –**

– apply a well padded splint between the limbs, and an additional long padded splint to the side of the fractured limb, extending from the armpit to the foot. Immobilise with two bandages round –

– the chest, just below the armpits;

– the pelvis, in line with the hip joints;

– together with five bandages, as described above, using a total of seven bandages.

One of the bandages may, in some instances, have to be omitted in order to avoid pressure over the site of the fracture.

Knee-cap (patella)

A fracture may be the result of muscular action which causes the bone to snap in two. It may also be fractured by direct force.

Treatment

1. Lay the casualty on his back with head and shoulders raised and supported (semi-recumbent position).

2. Raise and support the injured limb to a comfortable position.

3. Apply a splint along the back of the limb, reaching from the buttock to beyond the heel.

131

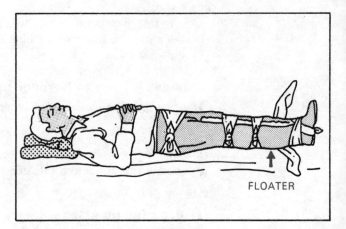

Figure 128: Treatment of casualty with fracture of lower limb: long or rough journey without splints

FLOATER

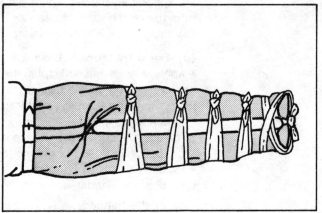

Figure 129: Long or rough journey with splints for lower limb

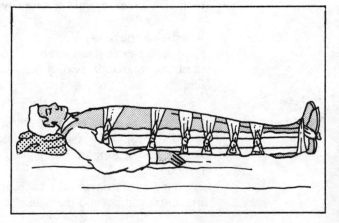

Figure 130: Long or rough journey with splints for thigh

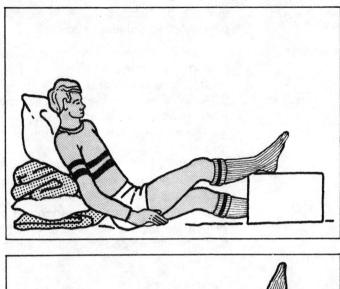

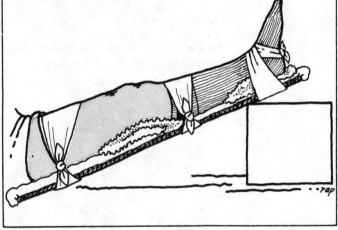

4. Place adequate soft padding under the natural hollow of the ankle, so as to raise the heel from the splint.

5. Secure the splint by the application of three bandages –

(*i*) figure-of-eight round ankle and foot;

(*ii*) broad bandage round the thigh;

(*iii*) broad bandage round the lower leg.

6. Keep the injured limb supported in a raised position.

Foot and toes – crushed foot

Commonly caused by a heavy weight dropping on or going

over the foot. A fracture should be suspected when there is pain, swelling and loss of power.

Treatment

1. Carefully remove shoe or boot and sock or stocking, cutting if necessary.
2. Treat a wound, if present.
3. Apply a well-padded splint to the sole of the foot, reaching from the heel to the toes.
4. Secure the splint with a figure-of-eight bandage as follows:—
The centre of a broad bandage is placed on the sole of the foot, the ends are crossed over the instep and carried to the back of the ankle; cross them and bring them to the front of the ankle where they are crossed once more and pass them under the sole of the foot. Tie off over the splint.
5. Raise and support the foot in a comfortable position.

Transport

All casualties with fractures of the lower limbs must be transported by stretcher.

CHAPTER NINE

Injuries to muscles, ligaments and joints

Strain

A strain is the over-stretching of a *muscle*.

Signs and symptoms

Sudden sharp pain at the site of injury.
In the case of a limb, the muscle may swell and cause severe cramp.

Treatment

1. Place the casualty in the most comfortable position.
2. Steady and support the injured part.
3. Arrange for medical aid.

Sprain

A sprain occurs at a **joint** and is caused by the wrenching or tearing of the ligaments and tissues connected with the joint.

Signs and symptoms

Pain at the joint;
– swelling about the joint and later bruising;
– inability to use the joint without increasing the pain.

Treatment

1. Rest and support the joint in the most comfortable position for the casualty.
2. Carefully expose the joint.
3. Apply pressure over the joint by –
– surrounding it with a good layer of cotton wool, keeping it in position by a bandage tied firmly; *or*
– apply a cold compress to the joint.

If a sprain of the ankle occurs out-of-doors, do not remove the boot or shoe but give additional support by applying a figure-of-eight bandage over the boot or shoe.

Note: In all doubtful cases treat as a fracture.

135

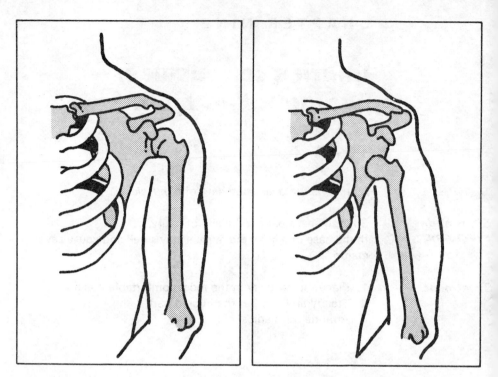

Figure 133: Normal shoulder   *Figure 134: Dislocation of the shoulder*

Dislocation

A dislocation is a displacement of one or more bones at a joint. The joints most frequently dislocated are those of the shoulder, elbow, thumb, fingers and lower jaw.

Signs and symptoms

Pain, severe and sickening in character, at or near the joint;
— abnormal appearance: deformity;
— fixity of the joint — casualty cannot move it;
— swelling and bruising are usually present.

In some cases it may prove difficult or even impossible for the First Aider to distinguish between a dislocation and a fracture: both may be present.

Treatment

1. Support and secure the part in the most comfortable position using pillow or cushion and bandages or slings.

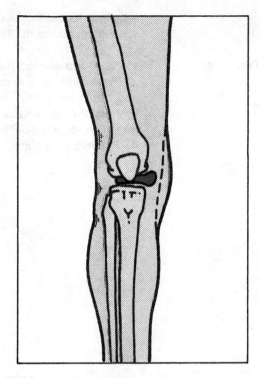

2. Obtain medical aid at once.
3. *Do not* attempt to replace the bones to a normal position.

Note: In all doubtful cases treat as a fracture.

Displaced cartilage of the knee (locked knee)

This occurs when a semi-lunar cartilage in the knee is displaced or torn, caused by, for example, a violent kick failing to connect at football, slipping on a step, twisting the body violently whilst standing on one leg.

Signs and symptoms

Pain, severe and sickening in character, referred to the inner side of the knee;
– the knee is held in a bent position; although it may be further flexed, it cannot be straightened;
– attempts to straighten the leg cause further severe pain;

137

– there is tenderness over the displaced cartilage;
– swelling, due to fluid in the joint, may occur.

Treatment

1. Raise and support the leg.
2. Protect the knee with soft padding extending well above and below the joint.
3. Keep the padding in position with a firm bandage in the most comfortable position for the casualty.
4. Remove to hospital.

CHAPTER TEN

The nervous system and unconsciousness

The nervous system

This consists of two parts –
– the Cerebro-spinal system, and
– the Autonomic system.

These together control the movements and functions of the body and the level of consciousness.

Cerebro-spinal system

This is made up of the brain, spinal cord and nerves. It enables sensations to be received and understood and allows action to be taken subsequently by the voluntary muscles (muscles under control of the will).

The **brain,** situated within the skull, is the seat of the intellect, the emotions and the will. It is here that impressions received by the senses (sight, hearing, touch, pain, etc.) and brought by the *sensory* nerves are analysed, and from where orders are given through the *motor* nerves to the muscles.

The **spinal cord** consists of nerve tissues extending from the brain through an opening in the base of the skull and continuing downwards to the lower part of the spine, behind the vertebral bodies.

The **nerves** proceed in pairs from each side of the brain and spinal cord, and their branches can be traced throughout the body.

When a sensory nerve is severed there is loss of sensation, when a motor nerve is severed there is loss of power of movement, in that part of the body to which their branches are distributed.

Autonomic system

This consists of a network of nerves which control the involuntary muscles and regulate many vital functions of

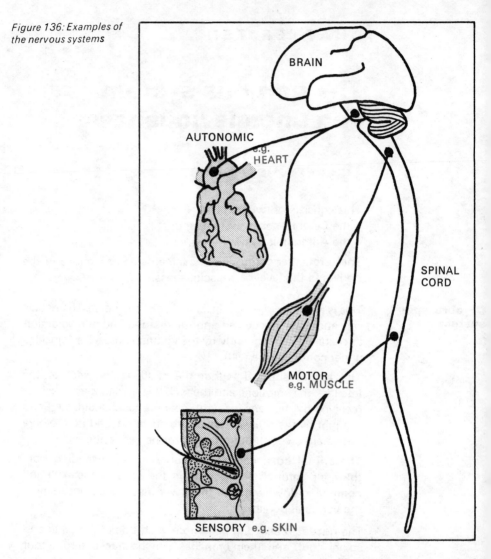

BRAIN

AUTONOMIC

e.g.
HEART

SPINAL
CORD

MOTOR
e.g. MUSCLE

SENSORY e.g. SKIN

the body. The autonomic system is not under the control of
the will and acts continuously, whether a person is awake or
asleep.

Unconsciousness

(*For examination of the unconscious casualty, see chapter 2*).

Unconsciousness is due to interruption of the normal

activity of the brain, brought about by some interference with the functions of the nervous system and circulation.

It may be progressive, and urgent treatment is therefore necessary.

Causes

These are numerous, but the most common are:

Asphyxia	Poisoning
Head injuries, with damage to the brain	Heart attacks
	Epilepsy
Shock	Infantile convulsions
Fainting	Diabetic emergencies
Stroke (apoplexy)	

Level of consciousness

The following terms are used for certain stages in a progression from consciousness to unconsciousness, or vice versa.

Full consciousness – alert, and able to answer questions normally.

Drowsiness – easily roused (e.g. gives normal answer to simple questions) but relapses into unconsciousness.

Stupor – can be roused only with difficulty. The casualty is aware of painful stimuli (e.g. nipping of the skin) but not of other external events (e.g. being spoken to); any answers may be unreliable.

Coma – cannot be roused at all.

These stages will help a First Aider to assess and quickly record changes in either direction.

Unless the casualty is fully alert, or can be roused easily, he should be treated as unconscious. It will be important for the doctor to know whether the onset of unconsciousness was sudden or slow.

General treatment

The aim of First Aid is to ensure an open airway and to obtain urgent medical attention.

1. (*a*) Make sure that the air passages are not obstructed; remove false teeth; clear the mouth of mucus, blood, vomit and any detached teeth – using a handkerchief when necessary. Loosen clothing about neck, chest and waist.

(*b*) Ensure there is plenty of fresh air to breathe; open windows and doors, or remove casualty from harmful gases or contaminated atmosphere.

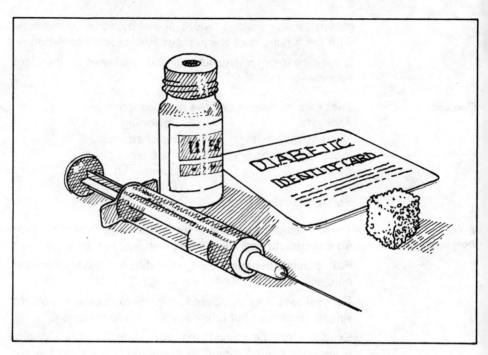

Figure 137: Insulin bottle; syringe; identity card; sugar

2. If breathing begins to fail or stop, immediately start artificial respiration.

3. When breathing is satisfactory and any severe bleeding controlled, establish level of consciousness, noting subsequently any change; check size of pupils and their reaction to light. Record this information for the doctor.

4. Dress wounds, immobilise limb fractures and place the casualty carefully in the recovery position with head slightly lower than the feet – so allowing secretions or vomit to drain away from the mouth.

5. His head should be pressed backward and his lower jaw pushed forward so that the chin juts out – thus preventing his tongue from blocking the back of the throat and choking him.

6. Cover with a blanket and place one under him if possible.

7. Make arrangements for transport to hospital in the recovery position.

142

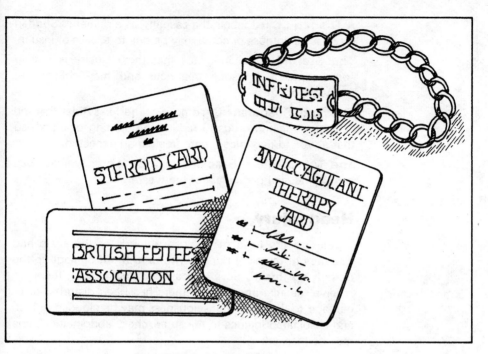

Figure 138: Steroid card; anti-coagulant card; epilepsy card, medic-alert bracelet

8. If removal to hospital is delayed, check the casualty's responses and pulse rate at intervals and keep a written record for the doctor.

9. If consciousness returns, speak reassuringly to the casualty; moisten his lips with water; if he is restless prevent him from hurting himself.

Do not give a drink to an unconscious casualty.

Do not leave him unattended.

Note: **Advise** any person who has been unconscious even for a moment to see his own doctor.

Further notes on the unconscious casualty

When examining an unconscious casualty make a search for a treatment card at the earliest opportunity in the presence of a reliable witness. It may be valuable in diagnosis.

143

A **Diabetic Card** labels the casualty as a diabetic. Sudden dizziness, faintness or coma may be due to excess of insulin.

The Steroid Card indicates that the casualty is having some form of cortisone treatment and may collapse in moments of stress.

The Anti-Coagulant Card notifies the First Aider that the casualty is taking drugs to reduce the clotting of blood, so that a wound may bleed more freely than expected.

The Medic-Alert Bracelet may be worn, which gives certain medical particulars of the wearer.

Head injury

Injuries to the head may cause wounds of the scalp and fractures of the skull bones, with or without damage to the underlying brain. Severe scalp wounds must therefore receive medical attention. If there has been disturbance or damage to the brain, consciousness may be clouded or lost, and associated injuries to the spine, chest, abdomen or limbs may be masked.

Many head injuries would be avoided if correct precautions were observed, such as the use of seat belts (see Chapter 14).

Fracture of the skull

See 'Injuries to Bones', page 111.

Injury to the brain

The brain like any other tissue may be damaged; such damage may result in cerebral concussion or compression.

Concussion

A condition of widespread but temporary disturbance of the working of the brain. 'Brain shaking' is a good description of what occurs. It may be caused by a blow on the head, a fall from a height on to the feet, falling heavily on the lower part of the spine, or a blow on the point of the jaw.

Signs and symptoms

Partial or complete loss of consciousness, lasting usually for a short time;
— breathing is shallow;
— shock is also present, so the casualty's face is pale, the skin cold and clammy, and the pulse rapid and weak;
— recovery may be accompanied by nausea and vomiting;

144

– loss of memory for events immediately before and after the injury is common.

Note: Should unconsciousness persist, suspect compression.

Compression

A condition of actual pressure on some part of the brain, by blood or fluid within the skull, or by a depressed fracture of the skull itself.

The condition may directly follow concussion with no return to consciousness, or it may develop some hours after apparent recovery.

Signs and symptoms

Most of the following will usually be present, but the absence of any of them does not rule out a diagnosis of compression.

Unconsciousness – coma may be present from the outset, particularly with actual damage to the brain tissue, or it may follow a period of stupor;

– in the early stages irritation of the brain may cause twitching of the limbs or even convulsions;

– the casualty's breathing becomes noisy;

– the body temperature may be raised with face flushed, and the pulse will become slow;

– the pupils of the eyes will be abnormal. They may –

– become unequal in size;

– both be dilated; *or*

– not react to light.

Weakness or paralysis on one side of the body may be present.

As compression develops, the casualty's alertness and level of consciousness fall; this change signifies the *most urgent need for medical care.*

Treatment

Concussion and Compression:
Carry out the general treatment of unconsciousness as far as is required.

In the case of concussion, keep careful watch for signs of compression developing.

Stroke (apoplexy)

This is due either to bleeding from a ruptured blood vessel into the brain, or the clotting *(thrombosis)* in a blood vessel of the brain. The condition usually occurs in middle-aged or elderly people suffering from high blood pressure; in a younger person, it is due to a weakness in the vessel wall from birth.

Signs and symptoms

These may vary from those of a somewhat less serious nature (sudden loss of power or sensation in a limb, or slurred speech) to serious signs of brain damage.

The sudden onset of the condition, the absence of history or signs of injury, and in some cases the age of the casualty, will help with diagnosis.

Confusion with acute alcoholic poisoning may arise but remember the casualty may have had or been given an alcoholic drink.

Treatment

Carry out the general treatment of unconsciousness so far as is required.

Epilepsy

This condition may occur at any age, but usually first appears in young people. Persons with epilepsy are liable to recurrent attacks, which may be of two types, minor and major; the latter may also be due to an addict taking an overdose of a stimulant drug.

Minor epilepsy

The individual becomes pale with eyes fixed and staring, and is not conscious of his surroundings.
He may then resume his previous activity as though nothing has happened.
The condition may resemble a fainting attack and should be treated as such.
If the person is known to be subject to such attacks, watch should be kept for the presence of post-epileptic automatism, described under Major Epilepsy.

Major epilepsy

This is a true epileptic fit.
The person sometimes has a premonition that he is going to have a fit. He may experience a sense of strangeness, accompanied by a headache, irritability, restlessness or a feeling of lethargy – the 'dreamy state'. These sensations, if they occur, are quite brief.

146

The fit consists of four stages –

(*i*) The casualty suddenly loses consciousness and falls to the ground, sometimes with a cry.

(*ii*) He remains rigid for a few seconds, during which time his face and neck becomes congested and cyanosed.

(*iii*) Convulsions, consisting of alternate contraction and relaxation of groups of muscles, begin. There is noisy breathing through a clenched jaw. Froth sometimes comes from the mouth and will be blood-stained if the tongue is bitten. He may lose control of the bladder and bowel and pass urine and motions involuntarily (incontinence).

(*iv*) The casualty then reaches the stage in which his muscles become relaxed (flaccid).

On regaining consciousness, he has loss of memory for recent events and may be dazed and confused and need a little while to gather himself together. He may act in a strange way and wander about without realising what he is doing (post-epileptic automatism); this condition varies in duration. Subsequently, he may feel exhausted and fall into a deep sleep.

Treatment
The aim of First Aid is to prevent the casualty, who has no control of himself, from receiving any injury, and to keep his airway clear.

1. Restrain the casualty only as far as is necessary. Forcible restraint of an epileptic may cause injury. Guide, but do not restrict, his movements.

2. Protect him from danger – fire, water, any object against which he might injure himself.

3. As opportunity arises, remove any false teeth and put a knotted handkerchief or similar soft material between his jaws, as far back as possible, to prevent his tongue being bitten. *Do not* try to prise open his mouth.

4. Wipe away any froth from the mouth.

5. Apply the general treatment of unconsciousness as far as is required.

6. Keep careful watch for a possible recurrence, and do not leave him until you are satisfied that he is fully aware of his surroundings.

7. Advise him to see his doctor, or if necessary, send him to hospital.

Do not arouse the casualty if he has fallen into a deep sleep.

Hysterical fits

These fits usually occur as a reaction to emotional upset or mental stress.

The attack may closely simulate an epileptic fit but is more dramatic and is staged to appeal to a sympathetic audience. The fit varies from a temporary loss of control, during which the person may shout and scream to a more dramatic effort with arms flying, crying, tearing at the hair or clothes, or rolling on the ground, etc., but taking care not to injure himself.

Treatment
1. Reassure the casualty gently but firmly.
2. As soon as possible give him something to do.
3. He should be kept under observation and considered as one in need of medical advice, when sufficiently recovered.

Convulsions in infants and young children

These sometimes occur as the result of a raised temperature from any cause, such as the onset of an infectious disease, throat or ear infection.

Signs and symptoms
There may be twitching of muscles of the face and limbs;
– occasional squinting or upturned eyes;
– there may be stiffness or rigidity, with the head and spine arched backwards, and holding of the breath;
– congestion of the face and neck;
– froth may appear at the mouth.

Treatment
1. Ensure a good supply of fresh air.
2. Loosen tight clothing about neck, chest and waist.
3. Place the child in the recovery position; if this is not possible, lay him down with head low and turned to one side.
4. If the child has a high temperature, this may be reduced by tepid sponging.
5. Obtain medical aid.
6. Reassure the child's parents.

Diabetes

Diabetes Mellitus (sweet or sugar diabetes) is the result of a disturbance of the normal method of using sugar supplies in the body because an internally produced substance from the pancreas (sweetbread) is insufficient. This substance is called *Insulin*.

Insulin or other drugs are prescribed for a diabetic in a quantity sufficient to keep the blood sugar at normal level. The danger for a diabetic under treatment with insulin is that of having more insulin than he needs, because –
—excessive exercise has already used up the sugar;
—insufficient food has been eaten, e.g. a meal has been delayed or missed, *or*
—the person may accidentally have given himself too much insulin.

Insulin coma Due to excess insulin.

Signs and symptoms
Pallor;
– profuse sweating;
– rapid pulse;
– shallow breathing – the breath is odourless;
– the limbs may tremble;
– confused – sometimes abnormally aggressive, or may appear to be drunk;
– faintness or unconsciousness: this develops quickly.

Warning: The longer a diabetic has been on insulin treatment, the less evident do any warning symptoms become to him.

Diabetic coma Due to an inadequate supply of insulin.

Signs and symptoms
Dry skin;
– face flushed;
– breathing deep. and sighing – breath smells strongly of musty apples or nail varnish (acetone);
– casualty passes gradually into a diabetic coma.

There may be uncertainty as to whether the casualty is suffering from excess or lack of insulin.

Treatment
1. **If conscious** (the casualty can confirm that he is a diabetic) –
– don't hesitate; give drink sweetened with two full table-

149

spoons of sugar, or give lumps of sugar, or other sweet substance.

If he improves dramatically, the problem has been one of excess of insulin; see that he gets more sugar in case he relapses into a coma.

If he does not improve, the giving of sugar will not cause any harm.

2. If unconscious –
– place in the recovery position.
Arrange for urgent admission to hospital.

Note: The casualty should be searched for a card indicating that he is a diabetic, and for lumps of sugar which are often carried by diabetics on insulin treatment. Marks of recent injections in the arm, thigh, or abdomen may be present.

CHAPTER ELEVEN

Burns and scalds

The effects of burns or scalds are similar and their seriousness depends upon many factors, the most important being the area and extent rather than the depth of the injury. However, in young children, especially infants, even small burns should be regarded as serious and hospital treatment sought without delay. The importance of adequate preventive measures cannot be over-emphasised.

The area of most burns and scalds, including the clothing involved, is usually sterile initially and every effort should be made to keep it sterile.

Types of injury

Superficial – a burn or scald where only the outer layers of the skin are damaged.

Deep – when the whole thickness of the skin, including the nerve endings, is destroyed.

An extensive superficial burn or scald is more painful than a small deep burn.

Burns

Burns are caused by –
– **dry heat** : such as fire, flame, contact with hot objects, exposure to sun;
– **electricity** : an electric current, or by lightning;
– **friction** : contact with a revolving wheel (brush burn), or a rope or wire;
– **corrosive chemicals** –
– *from acids* such as sulphuric, nitric, hydrochloric;
– *from alkalis* such as caustic soda, caustic potash, ammonia solution, quicklime;
– *from other chemicals* such as phosphorus, phenol (carbolic acid);
– **radiation** from X-ray overdose.

Scalds

Scalds are caused by –
– **moist heat** such as boiling water, a poultice applied too hot, steam, hot oil or tar.

Signs and symptoms

Pain – may be intense, especially with superficial burns;
– **redness** and later swelling and sometimes blistering, in severe cases charring;
– **shock;** there is great danger from shock which is directly related to the extent of the injury and increases rapidly with the loss of fluid (plasma) oozing from the burnt surface, and from the escape of blood or plasma into the tissues causing swelling.

Treatment of burns and scalds

The aim of First Aid is to reduce the local effects of heat; to relieve pain; to prevent infection of the affected area; to replace fluid loss and so lessen shock; and to remove a severely burned or scalded casualty to hospital as quickly as possible.

1. Lessen the spread of heat in the tissues and alleviate pain by placing the part gently under slowly running water or by immersing the part in cool water, keeping it there for at least ten minutes or until the pain ceases. At this early stage reduction of heat is essential, the risk of added infection being of lesser importance.
2. Remove promptly anything of a constrictive nature – rings, bangles, belts and boots, before the parts start to swell.
3. Clothing soaked in boiling water should be carefully removed. Cooled dry burned clothing already sterilised by heat need not be removed.
4. Lay the casualty down.
5. Cover the injured part with a dressing, clean sheet, pillow case, etc. With a burn of the face it may be necessary to cut a mask with a hole for breathing.
6. Immobilise a badly burned limb.
7. Give small cold drinks at frequent intervals to a badly burned casualty, if conscious.
8. Arrange for the immediate removal to hospital of all badly burned or scalded casualties as soon as possible, by stretcher if available.

9. Reassurance of the casualty is of great importance at all stages.

Do not apply any lotions, ointments or oil dressings.

Do not prick blisters, breathe or cough over, or touch the burned area, thereby increasing the risk of infection.

Clothing on fire

Action

Exclude air immediately to stop combustion

When a person's clothing catches fire, the immediate need is to remove the heat. Quench the flames and cool the tissues with water or other non-flammable fluid immediately to hand.

If no such fluid is immediately available, approach the person, holding a rug, blanket or coat, in front of yourself for protection, wrap it round him, lay him flat, and so smother the flames, by excluding air. *On no account should nylon or other such material be used.*

If a person's clothing catches fire when he is alone, he should roll himself on the floor smothering the flames with the nearest available wrap. On no account should he rush into the open air.

Burns or scalds of mouth or throat

May occur in children through drinking hot water from the spout of a kettle, or in suicide cases from swallowing a corrosive chemical. The taking of liquids which are too hot may also cause scalds.

The condition is very serious as there is much swelling of the tissues within the throat and this may interfere with breathing.

Treatment

1. Arrange for urgent removal to hospital.
2. Lay casualty down in recovery position.
3. If breathing is failing, give artificial respiration.
4. If conscious, give sips of cold water to drink.

Injuries from corrosive chemicals

In all cases speed is essential to prevent further damage.

153

Treatment

1. Flood the part thoroughly and continuously with running water if immediately available in order to dilute and eliminate the chemical. Avoid further damage to the burned tissues by using slowly running water. Make sure that the water drains away freely and safely.

2. Remove contaminated clothing carefully, if possible while flooding the injured part, taking precautions against contaminating yourself.

3. Continue treatment as for a burn.

4. Arrange urgent removal to hospital.

Note: Specific antidotes are normally available in industry as appropriate.

Eye injury from corrosive chemical

An eye may be injured by splashes of a liquid chemical or by solid matter such as lime.

The casualty complains of intense pain and intolerance of light. Urgent treatment is required.

Treatment

The aim of First Aid is to dilute and eliminate the chemical by flooding the eye immediately and copiously with the nearest available bland fluid, which will usually be water, even if it means soaking the casualty's clothing; to get the casualty to hospital.

1. (*a*) Hold the casualty's head under a gently running tap, or plunge it into a basin or a bucket of water and get him to blink his eye repeatedly.

(*b*) Sit or lay the casualty down, with head tilted right back and turned towards the affected side; protect the uninjured eye; flush the part copiously with tepid or cool water, gently opening the eyelids with your fingers.

Clean milk, if available, may be used initially.

2. If a solid corrosive chemical (such as lime) has entered the eye, rinse the upper lid and make sure that none is adhering to its surface.

3. Apply a dressing lightly over the eye.

4. **Arrange urgent removal to hospital.**

Special corrosives

Phosphorus: Yellow phosphorus ignites on exposure to air, as when drying on the skin.

Treatment

1. Keep the area flooded with water.

2. Apply a dressing soaked in water and ensure that it is always wet.
3. **Arrange urgent removal to hospital.**

Phenol (carbolic acid): Unless it is quickly removed, its corrosive and deeply penetrative action into the tissue will continue.

Treatment
1. Promptly remove all contaminated clothing.
2. Rub the skin for ten minutes with swabs soaked in water.
3. Apply a dressing.
4. **Arrange urgent removal to hospital.**

Electrical contact burns

These burns are normally found at those places of the body where the current entered and left the body.

The effect of the passage of an electric current through the body may be extremely severe and cause stoppage of breathing and heart action — requiring immediate treatment. Muscle spasm may throw the casualty away from the point of contact and cause other injuries such as broken bones.

The actual depth of the burn is likely to be greater than it appears, with damage to underlying tissues, although its area is relatively small.

If the casualty is not thrown clear, he may be fixed to the point of contact and receive extremely severe local burns.

Lightning may produce effects similar to those of an electrical injury. Patches of scorching may occur on the skin.

Treatment
1. If necessary give emergency resuscitation.
2. Treat as a burn.

Sunburn

Direct exposure of the skin to the sun's rays may produce itching and burning and redness, due to the dilatation of the blood vessels in the skin, or even superficial burns of the unacclimatised skin before a protective tan has developed. It can also be caused by sun-bathing with the body wet with sea water or sweat.

155

It may also arise in conditions of ice or snow or of desert sand, when the severity is increased by the reflection of ultra-violet radiations from these surfaces.

If the heat has been excessive, swelling and blistering may occur even after a short exposure. The head should be protected to prevent heat stroke.

Prevention of sunburn is by very gradual exposure of the skin to the sun in order to obtain a tan. In severe conditions, not more than five minutes exposure on the first day.

Treatment
1. Rest in the shade.
2. Give cold drink.
3. If sunburn is severe, seek medical aid.

Immersion of the part in cool water may have a soothing effect.

Note: Various skin lotions and creams are available for slight irritations or redness of the skin.

CHAPTER TWELVE

Poisoning

A poison is any substance, solid, liquid or gas, which, when taken into the body in sufficient amounts, may damage health or even destroy life.

It may be taken either accidentally or intentionally –
– *through the lungs* – breathing poisonous gases or fumes;
– *by the mouth* – swallowing;
– *by injection* – under the skin;
– *by absorption* – through the skin.

Through the lungs

This occurs mainly by breathing household gas (not North Sea Gas) fumes from fires, stoves, motor exhausts or smoke. Poisoning from industrial gases may also occur, e.g. carbon tetrachloride (contained in some fire extinguishers and dry cleaning solvents), trichorethylene (present in de-greasing and dry cleaning agents), is also employed as an anaesthetic. Hydrogen sulphide, cyanogen gas or cyanide fumes are rapidly fatal.

By the mouth

Swallowed poisons act quickly, *either* –
– **directly on the food passage** causing retching, vomiting, pain, and often diarrhœa. *Common causes* are poisonous berries and infected and decomposed food. Severe symptoms are caused by corrosives (strong acids and alkalis) which burn the lips, mouth, gullet and stomach and cause intense pain.
Or—
– **on the nervous system** after absorption into the blood. *Common causes* are excessive alcohol, tablets and solutions taken to relieve pain (aspirin, preparations containing opium derivatives) or to produce sleep (barbiturate drugs). A few poisons act on the nervous system causing delirium (e.g. belladonna) or fits (e.g. strychnine, prussic acid).

By injection under the skin

These arise from bites of poisonous reptiles, some animals and certain insects, or by hypodermic syringe, e.g. deliberate taking of drugs, such as heroin.

By absorption through the skin

Common causes are certain pesticides used by farmers (such as parathion malathion etc.). They cause convulsions if swallowed.

Warning: Apart from the possibility of death, life may be endangered by :–

– *asphyxia:* which may occur from the results of poisons especially those taken through the lungs or acting on the nervous system ;

– *convulsions:* which may occur as a result of poisons absorbed through the skin ;

– *coma:* which may occur from the results of the poisons in any group.

General rules for treatment of poisoning

The aim of First Aid is to sustain life and remove the casualty urgently to hospital.

1. If the casualty is conscious –
– ask him quickly what happened ; remember he may lose consciousness at any time.

If lips and mouth show signs of burns give quantities of water, milk or barley water to dilute the poison.
Remove the casualty to hospital quickly by car or ambulance.

– If casualty is unconscious –
– *if breathing freely*, place him in the recovery position, thus ensuring an open airway ;
– *if breathing is failing or has ceased*, commence artificial respiration immediately. This may have to be continued until hospital treatment can be given, as part of the breathing mechanism has been disturbed by the poison.
Remove the casualty to hospital quickly by ambulance.

2. Send any particulars of the suspected cause, if known, to hospital with the casualty, together with –
– any remaining poison ;

— any box, carton, bottle or other container which may help to identify the poison;
— any vomited matter.

Note: Suicides often take all the tablets and dispose of the containers.

Additional treatment for special cases of poisoning

Industrial gas

Do not attempt to rescue unless equipped with, and practised in the use of, a respirator and a life line.

Pesticides

The casualty must not be allowed to exert himself at all.
1. Remove contaminated clothing.
2. If convulsions present, treat as a fit.
3. Sponge freely with cold water his head, back of neck, spine and body.
4. Place him in a current of air; if necessary fan him.
5. Give as much water or well sweetened drink as he can swallow.

Rat Poison

These food baits are highly poisonous and dangerous to children.
Send to hospital any child who has eaten these baits.

Notes on some common poisons

Sudden illness associated with the taking of drugs or other unusual substances should be referred to a doctor.

Barbiturates and other sleeping tablets: There is respiratory depression with failure of breathing, leading to collapse or even coma, with failure of circulation and kidney function.

Alcohol: The casualty smells of alcohol, is in a confused state, co-ordination is poor, pupils are dilated, sleepiness, collapse or coma will ensue.

Note: Barbiturate plus alcohol is a most dangerous combination of poisons. **Take the casualty to hospital immediately.**

Aspirin: The casualty has pain in the abdomen, nausea, depression, drowsiness, or coma, sweating profusely with

159

laboured breathing and full pulse.

Aspirin is a constituent of most pain reducing tablets, influenza and cold remedies. An excessive dose may be taken deliberately by adults but accidentally by children.

Iron or anaemia tablets: These attract children because of their attractive colour and sweet taste. Overdose causes retching and vomiting, often blood-stained. The casualty is cold, drowsy and restless, pulse rapid.

Travel sickness tablets: Atropine-like drugs. Cause excitement initially, depression later.

Belladonna (Deadly Nightshade) contains atropine. Children are attracted by the ripe coloured berries in the autumn, and eating such berries causes the skin to be hot and flushed. Temperature rises to 40°C (104°F). The mouth is dry and there is intense thirst. The pupils are widely dilated and breathing is noisy. The casualty may be excitable in the early stages but depressed later.

Laburnum pods: These cause burning in mouth and abdomen; nausea, severe vomiting; diarrhoea or collapse; delirium; twitching; unconsciousness.

Petroleum products: The ingestion of these substances is becoming more common, especially with children. Although there will be no burn marks, on no account should attempts be made to induce vomiting.

CHAPTER THIRTEEN

Miscellaneous conditions

Extremes of temperature

Excessive cold and heat can cause damage to the skin or body in such a way that tissues locally or body function generally may be so seriously affected that death results.
Locally, cold may cause frostbite at the extremities (fingers, toes, ears and nose), while heat can cause blistering and ulceration of exposed parts.

If the whole body is affected, the important factors determining the result, and the type of treatment to be given, are the age of the person affected and the degree of fatigue or exhaustion. The young adult after exposure to cold can be warmed up quickly, but care should be taken to heat an infant or elderly casualty gradually.

Effects of cold

Cold exhaustion This may be experienced by those on explorations, mountaineering, etc., especially under conditions of extreme cold. Wind, snow and rain exacerbate the effects. The onset is insidious and may pass unnoticed. The severity of reaction varies with age and the casualty's physical condition. These govern individual resistance. The healthy adult regulates his body temperature naturally, but if over-fatigued by exercise and anxiety may suffer from 'exposure' (the term often used to describe this condition).

Signs and symptoms
– Increasing slowness of physical and mental response;
– stumbling, cramps and shivering;
– slurring of speech and difficulty of vision;
– unreasonable behaviour or irritability;
– pulse and respiration increased at first, while the body can still respond to cold by shivering.

Warning to travellers: If any of these symptoms occur – **take shelter or improvise shelter, and rest.**

It is essential—
– to prevent further loss of body heat;
– to overcome exhaustion;
– to obtain help if possible.

If these precautions are *not* taken, the excessive cold will overcome the heat-regulating processes, the temperature falls, and the casualty will fall asleep from cold exhaustion. Temperature falls to about 25°C (77°F), breathing is depressed (slow and shallow) and the pulse rate is very slow. Death will result when the body temperature falls to about 20°C (68°F).

All severely affected cases should be placed in the recovery position and taken by stretcher to medical aid as quickly as possible, protecting them from cold during the journey.

Treatment

At the site:—
1. Protect the casualty from wind, rain or sleet, and from cold wet ground under him.
2. If possible, wrap him in dry clothing; put him in a sleeping bag.
3. Give warm drinks, e.g. condensed milk.

At base:—
Rapid rewarming in a hot bath, bringing the temperature up to 42°C–45°C (107°F–113°F).
Note: **All cases** of prolonged exposure to cold should be considered as serious and in urgent need of medical supervision.

Severe accidental cooling of the body (hypothermia)

This is a dangerous lowering of the body temperature which may occur at any age, but especially in babies and the elderly who lack the ability to regulate their own temperature, even when not fatigued. There is a loss of surface heat followed by cooling of the deep tissues and organs of the body.

Causes

– Exposure to cold – from weather or in an unheated home;

162

– prolonged immersion in cold water – e.g. shipwreck in Arctic or Antarctic conditions;
– lowering of sensibility to cold by alcohol, drugs or poisoning.

A contributory cause may be a medical condition, e.g. diabetes.

Infants: Babies must be kept constantly warm during the first few weeks of life as they cannot regulate their own body temperature.

Elderly and infirm: Those living alone, especially pensioners on an inadequate diet, may be found in a state of stupor on the floor or collapsed in an outside passage or lying unconscious in bed. In each case, they may be fully clothed.

This condition can easily be mistaken for a 'stroke' or heart attack.

Signs and symptoms

Infants are quiet and refuse food. Pink face, hands, and feet, if present, are deceptive.

Elderly and infirm are pale and in a state of collapse.
The casualty is deathly cold to the touch;
– the pulse is slow, weak or imperceptible;
– breathing is slow and shallow.

Treatment

The aim of First Aid in *all* cases is to prevent further heat loss, improve body heat and circulation, and to obtain medical aid or transport the casualty to hospital.

1. Place the casualty between blankets so that the body temperature can recover *gradually.*
2. If conscious, give tepid or warm, sweet drinks.

Do *not* use hot water bottles or electric blankets as this will cause sudden dilatation of the superficial blood vessels, taking away blood from the deep tissues and essential organs: this may cause a fatal collapse due to a drop in the casualty's blood pressure and temperature.

Frostbite

Most commonly occurs if a part of the body is exposed to the wind in very cold weather. The ears, nose, chin, fingers and toes are most frequently affected.

163

Signs and symptoms	The casualty may feel the affected part cold, painful and stiff; – feeling and power of movement may be lost; – blanching and numbness of the part is evident. In severe cases, if treatment is not urgently carried out, gangrene of the affected parts or death may occur.
Treatment	1. Take care of the casualty's general condition by sheltering him from the weather; give warm drinks. 2. Promptly remove anything of a constrictive nature – gloves, rings, boots. 3. Thaw the affected part – **face** – cover with a dry, gloved hand until normal colour and sensation return; **hands** – place under the clothing in his armpits; **feet** – wrap in a warm blanket or sleeping bag. 4. **Transport the casualty to medical aid as quickly as possible.** *Do not* rub the affected part. *Do not* apply direct heat in any form.

Effects of excessive heat

In persons who are not accustomed to high temperatures, *heat exhaustion* or *heat stroke* can occur.

Heat exhaustion	This is slow in onset and gives rise to a shocked condition due to a salt and water deficiency.
Causes	Exposure to excessive heat, especially moist heat, and is commonly found in newcomers to very hot climates. Fluid and salt loss is considerable from excessive sweating and is often aggravated further by a gastrointestinal upset with diarrhœa and vomiting. A person who is acclimatised to the tropics may also be affected by water deficiency following a severe attack of malaria or other tropical fever.
Signs and symptoms	Muscular cramp from salt deficiency is an early sign; – the casualty is exhausted and may be restless; – the face is pale and cold and has a clammy sweat; there may be sudden collapse and loss of consciousness; – pulse and breathing are rapid;

164

− temperature may be normal, sub-normal, or slightly elevated;
− a complaint of headaches, dizziness and nausea, and sometimes of abdominal cramp, may be made;
− sudden movement may cause fainting (*syncope*).

Treatment

1. Place and keep the casualty in cool surroundings.
2. If conscious, give cold water to drink. If casualty has had excessive sweating, cramps or diarrhœa and/or vomiting, add half a teaspoonful of common salt to each pint (half a litre) of water.
3. Obtain medical aid.

Heat stroke

The onset is more sudden and may be preceded by heat exhaustion.

Causes

May be brought on by a high atmospheric temperature, with a hot, drying wind or by a high humidity and lack of air current. It may also be caused by malaria or other debilitating illness. The body can no longer control its temperature by sweating.

Signs and symptoms

Unconsciousness may come on quickly. A temperature of 40°C (104°F) or more may occur;
− the casualty is restless, and, if conscious, complains of headache, dizziness and feeling hot;
− face is flushed, the skin hot and dry to the touch;
− pulse is full and bounding;
− breathing is noisy;
− there may be confusion or stupor, and coma may result.

Treatment

The aim of First Aid is to reduce the casualty's temperature as quickly as possible.

1. Strip the casualty and wrap in a wet, cold sheet: keep it wet until the casualty's temperature has been lowered to 38°C (101°F).
2. Place him in the recovery position.
3. Direct currents of air on to the casualty from above and below by hand or by electric fans.
4. On recovery, the casualty, with a dry sheet over him, should be transported into air-conditioned accommodation to prevent relapse.
5. If his temperature rises again, repeat the treatment.
6. Send to hospital.

Cramp

This is defined as sudden, involuntary and painful contraction of a muscle or group of muscles.

Causes

Poor muscular co-ordination during exercise;
– chilling, as in swimming;
– excessive loss of salt and body fluids from severe sweating, diarrhœa, or persistent vomiting.

Treatment

The shortened muscles must be stretched.

In the hand: Forcibly, but gently, straighten out the fingers.
In the thigh: Straighten the knee and raise the leg with one hand under the heel while pressing down the knee with the other hand.

In the calf or foot: Straighten the knee, and with the hand forcibly draw the foot up towards the shin; *or –*
straighten the toes and get the casualty to stand on the ball of the foot.

Salt deficiency: give copious drafts of cold water to which has been added a half teaspoonful of salt to a pint (half a litre) of water.

The eye

All eye injuries are potentially serious, and blows by blunt objects may damage not only the eyelids and the exposed part of the eye but also rupture blood vessels of the eye, the lens and the retina.

Any wounds caused by sharp tools, or even tiny particles which may perforate the eyeball, are potentially serious because of damage which they do mechanically, chemically and by the infection which they may produce.

For all serious injuries to the eye, *immediate medical aid is indicated.*

Foreign body in the eye

Particles of grit, loose eyelashes, small fragments of metal or glass, etc. may lodge on the eyeball or under the eyelid causing considerable discomfort and inflammation if not speedily removed.

Treatment

1. Prevent the casualty from rubbing the eye.

166

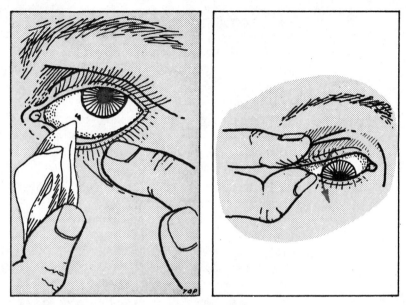

Figures 139 and 140: Removal of foreign body from the eye

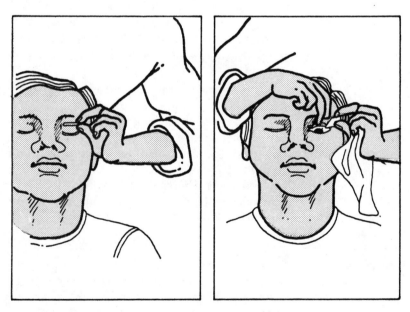

Figures 141 and 142: Removal of foreign body from the eye

2. *Do not* attempt to remove the foreign body if it is –
– on the pupil of the eye; *or*
– embedded or adherent to the eyeball; *or*
– cannot be seen but the eye is inflamed and painful.

The following treatment should be given –
(*i*) Close the eyelids.
(*ii*) Cover the eye with a soft pad of cotton wool, extending to forehead and cheek, and secure lightly in position with a bandage.
(*iii*) Obtain medical aid.

3. If the foreign body can be seen and is neither on the pupil nor adherent to the eyeball –
(*i*) seat the casualty facing the light, stand in front of him and pull down the lower lid;
(*ii*) then remove the foreign body with the corner of a clean handkerchief or a wisp of cotton wool which has been soaked in a little water.

4. If the foreign.body is under the upper lid, ask the casualty to look down, grasp the eyelashes and pull the upper lid downwards and outwards over the lower lid. The foreign body may thus be dislodged by the lashes of the lower lid. If not, ask the casualty to blink his eye under water.

If still unsuccessful and medical aid is not immediately available –
(*i*) stand behind the casualty, steadying his head against your chest, and ask him to look down;
(*ii*) place a smooth matchstick at the base of the upper lid and press it gently backwards;
(*iii*) grasp the lashes and turn the lid over the matchstick, so everting the eyelid;
(*iv*) remove the foreign body with the corner of a clean handkerchief or a wisp of cotton wool which has been soaked in a little water.

Injury to the eyeball

The eye may be involved in a wound or a crush injury.

Treatment

1. Lay the casualty down at absolute rest.
2. Close the lid and cover the eye with a soft pad of cotton wool, extending to forehead and cheek. Apply a bandage lightly.
3. Remove to hospital as soon as possible.

Acids and alkalis	**Strong acids or alkalis in the eye:** *For treatment of strong acids or alkalis in the eye see 'Injuries from corrosive chemicals', page 154.*

The ear

Foreign bodies in the ear canal	*Insects:* Flood the ear with tepid water or olive oil; the insect will float out. *Foreign bodies* (beads, beans, etc.): **Do not** attempt to remove these objects, but take the casualty (usually a small child) to a doctor or hospital.
Bleeding	If bleeding occurs from a laceration of the **outer ear** – – control by direct pressure over a dressing or other clean material and bandage in position, if necessary. If from the **ear canal** – – *after a head injury*, suspect a fracture of the skull. – *after a blow or blast involving the ear*, a rupture of the eardrum is likely.
Treatment	See 'Bleeding from special areas', page 93.
Earache	May occur suddenly during air travel or in underwater swimming, due to a sudden change of pressure on the drum. It may also occur through inflammation as in a head cold.
Treatment	1. *During air travel:* The casualty should try and equalise the pressure by – – holding his nose, and at the same time swallowing; *or* – blowing out the cheeks. 2. *Underwater swimming* – The same procedure can be carried out after the person has surfaced. 3. *Inflammation* – Do not attempt procedure in 1 above, but **obtain medical aid immediately.**

Toothache

In a persistent form, this can often cause distress and needs dental attention.

In the absence of dental aid, the application of warmth and oil of cloves to the offending tooth will often bring relief. The taking of a mild pain-relieving tablet may assist, but it is the casualty's own responsibility.

Headache

This is always a symptom of some other condition. It occurs frequently when the temperature rises or from eyestrain.

Headaches are often due to worry and stress and are usually relieved by reassurance and a mild pain-relieving tablet.

If it persists or occurs frequently, the casualty should see his own doctor.

Foreign body in the nose

Treatment
1. Instruct the casualty to breathe through his mouth.
2. Take the casualty (usually a small child) to a doctor.
Do not attempt to remove the foreign body.

Foreign body in the stomach

Pins and other small objects, such as coins or buttons, may accidentally be swallowed, especially by young children. Smooth objects need not necessarily cause alarm.

Treatment
1. Calm the casualty and parents.
2. Medical advice should be sought.
Do not give anything by the mouth.

Rupture (abdominal hernia)

This condition is a protrusion of some part of the abdominal contents through the muscular wall of the abdomen under the skin.

It occurs most frequently in the groin, but it is not uncommon at the navel or through the scar of an abdominal operation. It may occur after exercise, lifting heavy objects, coughing or even when straining on the lavatory when constipated.

The condition may arise as painless swelling, which may persist or worsen. It may occur suddenly with swelling, pain and possible vomiting. ('Strangulated' hernia may present these symptoms and signs and is an urgent surgical problem).

Treatment
1. Reassure the casualty.
2. Lay him down and support his head and shoulders, bend and support his knees;

– if vomiting occurs or seems likely, place him in the recovery position.
3. Seek medical aid if pain or vomiting persists.
Do not **attempt to reduce the swelling.**

Asthma

Sudden attacks of difficult breathing occur most often at night, and the casualty has difficulty in forcing air out of his lungs.

eatment

1. Place the casualty in a comfortable position, usually sitting up or leaning forward resting on a table or pillow, but keeping the back straight.
2. Reassure him and provide plenty of fresh air.
3. Obtain medical aid or send to hospital.

Hiccups

Commonly the result of a digestive disturbance or 'nervousness'.

Relief may be obtained in various ways, e.g. sips of water, holding the breath or distracting the attention.

If the condition persists for more than a few hours, the casualty's doctor should be informed.

Stings and bites

Vinegar for Wasp Stings
Bicarb of Soda for Bee stings.

tings

Bees, Hornets, Wasps

eatment

1. Remove the sting, if present, using forceps or tweezers or the point of a needle which has been sterilised by passing it through a flame and then cooling it.
2. Antihistamine creams are useful if applied immediately. Otherwise, apply surgical spirit or a weak ammonia solution or a solution of bicarbonate of soda.
3. If the sting is in the mouth, give a mouthwash of one teaspoonful of bicarbonate of soda to a tumbler of water. If there is much swelling in the mouth or if there is difficulty in breathing, place the casualty in the recovery position and give ice to suck. Seek medical aid immediately.

171

Bites

Dog bites

Treat as for a wound.

In countries where rabies may be present, all casualties suffering from dog bites should be referred to medical aid for special serum treatment.

Snake bites

Snakes will not usually attack unless stepped on or cornered.

Some snakes are poisonous and their bite is dangerous and may be fatal.

Snake bites are greatly feared, and the fear increases the degree of shock to the casualty. Many persons have died from fright after being bitten.

In those countries where dangerous snakes are common anti-snake serum is kept available in known centres. If the snake is killed, it should be kept for identification.

Treatment

1. Calm and reassure the casualty and lay him down. Never let him walk about if agitated.
2. Flush the wound with soapy water and wash away all venom that may be around the wound or has oozed from it
3. Support and immobilise the limb.
4. Obtain medical aid as soon as possible.
5. Should breathing begin to fail, commence artificial respiration.

'Winding'

The result of a blow in the upper part of the abdomen (*solar plexus*) which may cause fainting or even collapse.

Treatment

1. Place the casualty in the recovery position.
2. Loosen tight clothing at the neck, chest and waist.
3. Gently massage the upper abdomen.

Stitch

A painful spasm of the diaphragm. It occurs during games and running, particularly if the person is not in training, or if exercise is taken too soon after a meal.

Treatment

1. If not immediately relieved by rest, give sips of hot water
2. Gently rub the affected part of the abdomen.

172

CHAPTER FOURTEEN

Procedure at road accidents

The increase of traffic on the roads has, inevitably, brought about an increase in the number of accidents to pedestrians, other road users and to occupants of motor vehicles.

All categories may be injured in one accident. Some casualties, especially small children and babies, may be out of sight having been thrown some distance away, catapulted over a hedge or hidden by a rug within the vehicle.

If in your own car, park it in a safe place, preferably off the road, before attending to the accident.

Many injuries could be avoided by the use of suitable safety-belts, crash helmets and neck rests.

It should always be borne in mind that the damaged car, or one passing, may have a First Aid outfit, and a fire extinguisher may also be available.

Road accidents can be divided into three main categories:
1. Accidents involving those outside a vehicle (e.g. pedestrians, cyclists).
2. Accidents involving the occupants of vehicles.
3. Accidents involving both.

Many of the casualties who have died in such accidents might have been saved by correct early treatment, and every effort must be made to reduce the number of fatalities. These occur particularly between the time of the accident and the arrival at hospital.

In dealing with road accidents, the First Aider must ensure that no further danger is present or can occur. Accordingly, the following instructions are given which, if carried out, will lessen possible causes of further danger.

Immediate action

Protect the scene of the accident.
Do not run to the car and start pulling the injured out, which

173

is the usual instinctive action. If you do, you may easily kill injured persons who could be saved, or be killed yourself.

Stop a passing car and ask the driver to telephone emergency service required. Give the exact location of the accident, number of injured, and any other relevant information, such as trapped casualties.

Send someone to put out reflective warning triangles on both sides of the accident, commencing 200–400 yards or metres away. If you have no triangles flag down the traffic at this distance.

Much of this could be done by bystanders. The more they are given to do the less they will interfere.

Do not let well-meaning people bundle the injured into cars and rush them to hospital.

Calculated risk

In a motor accident there may be conditions when the calculated risk has to be taken.

The problems in these conditions are *when* and *how* to remove a casualty from a crashed vehicle when —
– a proper examination is difficult or impossible;
– he may be unconscious;
– he probably has multiple injuries.

The difficulty is how to know that an unconscious casualty has no spinal injury, unless he recovers consciousness. Therefore all unconscious casualties in crashed vehicles must be treated as if they had a fracture, i.e. leave them in the vehicle and do ***not*** attempt to move them unless the situation is dangerous, when it may be necessary. It is better, if possible, to leave spinal injuries or suspected spinal injuries until the Ambulance or Fire Brigade arrive.

It may be necessary to move an unconscious casualty quickly if —
– the heart or breathing stops. The First Aider should make every effort to keep the casualty's airway open.
– if the car is on fire or there is danger of explosion or fire.

Again, remember that conscious casualties with multiple injuries and much shock may not be complaining of, or suffering from, pain, and it will be necessary to ask whether they have numbness or tingling in arms or legs, remembering

174

that their information under these circumstances may not be reliable.

Accidents involving those outside a vehicle

As a general rule a First Aider *should* deal with a seriously injured casualty at the site of the accident.

Unnecessary movement may aggravate the casualty's condition and worsen the injuries. However, the safety and care of the casualty are of the greatest importance and if it is necessary to move the injured person urgently from the roadway it should be done *as carefully and as gently as possible.*

In the case of a pedestrian who is trapped under a car and has to be removed owing to the possibility of fire, the vehicle should be carefully immobilised by applying the hand brake, chocking the wheels with stones to prevent slipping and to ensure that the vehicle makes no un-controlled movement.

A note should be made of the exact position of the casualty, if moved, also the time and place of the accident as this information may be required by the police, who should be informed of all accidents.

Accidents involving occupants of vehicles

Switch off the engine; better still, disconnect the battery.
Apply the hand brake: use wheel chocks if necessary;
Do not allow smoking by anyone.

If a fire does not start right away it is unlikely to occur, except from a lighted match or perhaps cigarette of a thoughtless motorist. Fire in the wiring usually begins as smouldering under the bonnet or dashboard.

Do not remove the injured immediately, unless in danger;
Locate the fire, if any, from the smoke and attack

175

with a fire extinguisher, blanket or earth.

Treatment

Wherever possible leave the removal of severely injured casualties to the Emergency Services which have been specially trained to deal with such conditions.

If, however, it is essential to move the casualty, e.g. because of fire risk, etc., when possible ensure you have adequate help to support all parts of the casualty and aim to make the removal from the car in one continuous smooth operation.

The *priorities of treatment* in road accidents should be directed to:
(*i*) breathing;
(*ii*) bleeding;
(*iii*) unconsciousness.

If an unconscious casualty should not be moved, preparation should be made to facilitate rapid removal in the event of danger to the casualty being increased or suspicion of the heart or breathing ceasing. This will warrant the removal of such a casualty without awaiting further assistance from Ambulance or Fire Brigade Services.

Removal

To prepare casualty for rapid removal

It has been noticed that accident victims may be trapped by a foot being held under the car seat or piece of twisted metal, and cannot escape from the crashed vehicle. In such cases, quickly release the casualty and thus facilitate his removal from the crashed vehicle.

Injuries can be caused by people who attempt to lift a car and finding it impossible, allow the car to fall back again. The side of a car can be lifted but care should be taken not to push the other side of the car on to any bystanders.

If the casualty is conscious and can be reached he should be questioned and examined where he is, for bleeding and fractures. The former must be controlled and the latter immobilised by fixing the limbs to each other or to the trunk. If a neck injury is suspected, it is possible to improvise a neck collar by folding a newspaper or other suitable firm paper, if available, into 4 inch (10 centimetres) folds, placing it round the neck and retaining it in position with a bandage.

If the crashed car has a bucket seat, then an attempt should be made to remove the casualty in position on the seat, if possible.

Prepare for blanket lift by arranging a blanket concertina pattern and inserting under the knees. Pull out the top edge to back of seat under the casualty, easing him to permit this. Then draw the free edge up the back to the top of the shoulders taking care to avoid catching the edge in coat or overcoat.

Maintain observation on breathing and pulse.

Make the casualty comfortable, moving him as gently and as little as possible.

Reassure him and protect him from cold.

Ensure that all unconscious casualties are carried in the recovery position.

Trapped casualty

Impaired breathing in the trapped casualty

In many positions the tongue tends to fall to the back of the throat and block the airway. Push the jaw forward and have a handkerchief ready so the tongue can be drawn out after the mouth has been opened. Oxygen can be administered to a casualty in a car if suitable apparatus is available but emergency resuscitation cannot always be carried out until the casualty has been removed. In these circumstances the insertion of an airway by a Doctor, Nurse or Ambulance Attendant would be a valuable procedure.

Severe injuries involving the mouth

Where severe facial injuries involve the mouth in unconscious casualties, especially if the jaw is broken, it can be very difficult to maintain an adequate airway.

CHAPTER FIFTEEN

Handling and transport of injured persons

The comfort and well being of the casualty is the first consideration. His condition must not be aggravated nor his life jeopardised by frequent handling, or rough and hurried evacuation. If the casualty is seriously injured, or if he has multiple injuries, it may be better to deal with him where he lies, as much damage can be caused in removal. A First Aider acting alone, or with unskilled help, may easily cause more damage trying to move the casualty than by dealing with him at the site of the accident.

Before moving a casualty, unless life is endangered by fire, falling debris, or a poisoned atmosphere, it is important, especially if he is unconscious, to carry out a quick but systematic examination of the head and neck, chest and abdomen and all limbs which, if injured, must be supported during removal.

A sick or injured person may be removed to shelter by the following methods:–

1. Support by a single helper.
2. Handseats and the 'kitchen chair' carry.
3. Blanket lift.
4. Stretcher.
5. Wheeled transport (e.g. ambulance).
6. Air and sea transport.

The method to be adopted, and it may be necessary to use more than one, will depend upon –
(a) the nature and severity of the injury;
(b) the number of helpers and facilities available;
(c) the distance to shelter;
(d) the nature of the route to be travelled.

Treatment The aim of the First Aid treatment is to enable the

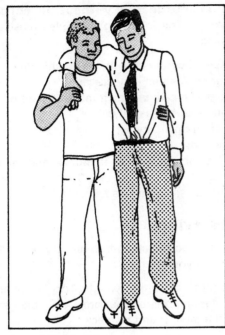

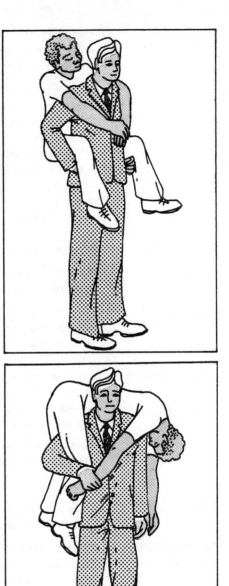

Figure 143 (above): Human crutch

Figure 144 (top right): Pick-a-back

Figure 145 (right): Fireman's lift and carry

casualty to reach his destination without his condition becoming worse. The following principles must be regularly kept in mind:—

1. The position assumed by the casualty or in which he has been placed, must not be altered unnecessarily.
2. Throughout transport a careful watch must be kept on —
— the general condition of the casualty;
— the maintenance of an open airway;
— the control of bleeding;
— the continuous immobilisation of fractures and large wounds.
3. The transport must be safe and steady.

Methods of carrying

Note: If help is available, do not attempt to move a seriously ill or injured casualty on your own.

Cradle

This is for casualties of light weight or children. Lift the casualty by passing one of your arms well beneath his two knees, and the other round his neck.

Human crutch

Standing at his injured side, except where there is injury to an upper limb, assist the casualty by putting your arm round his ·waist, grasping his clothing at his hip, and placing his arm round your neck, holding his hand with your free hand.

If his upper limbs are uninjured and his other hand is free, the casualty may gain additional help from a staff or walking stick.

Pick-a-back

If the casualty is conscious and able to hold on, he may be carried in the ordinary 'pick-a-back' fashion.

Fireman's lift and carry

Note: To be used only when the casualty is not too heavy. Help the casualty to rise to the upright position. Grasp his right wrist with your left hand. Bend down with your head under his extended right arm so that your right shoulder is level with the lower part of his abdomen, and place your right arm between or round his legs. Taking the weight on your right shoulder rise to the erect position. Pull the casualty across both shoulders and transfer his right wrist to your right hand, so leaving your left hand free.

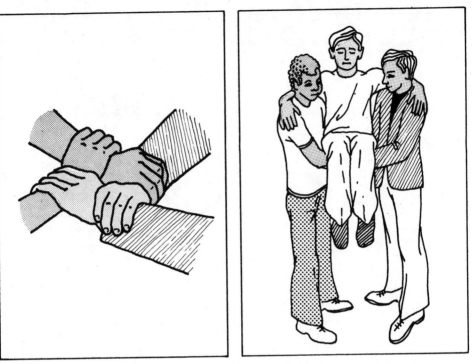

Figures 146 and 147: Four-handed seat

By two or more First Aiders

4-handed seat

This seat is used when the casualty can assist by using one or both arms.

Two First Aiders face each other behind the casualty and grasp their left wrists with their right hands and each others' right wrists with their left hands and stoop down.

The casualty is instructed to place one arm round the neck of each First Aider, so that he may raise himself to sit on their hands and steady himself during transport.

The First Aiders rise together and step off with outside feet and walk with ordinary paces forward.

2-handed seat

This seat is mostly used to carry a casualty who is unable to assist by using his arms.

Two First Aiders face each other and stoop one on each side of the casualty. Each First Aider passes his forearm nearest

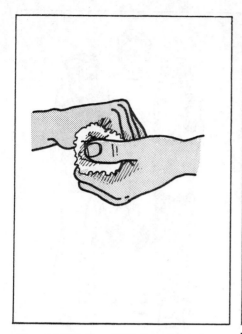

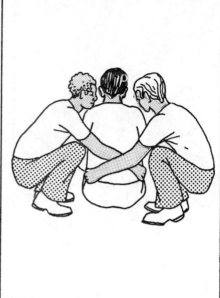

Figures 148, 149 and 150: Two-handed seat

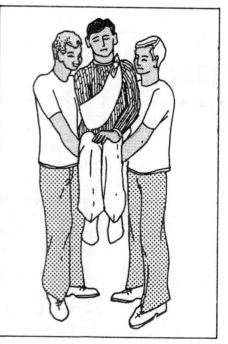

182

Figure 151: Kitchen chair method

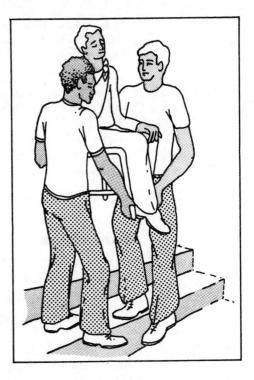

the casualty's body under his back just below the shoulders and, if possible, takes hold of clothing. They slightly raise the casualty's back and then pass their other forearms under the middle of his thighs and clasp their hands, the First Aider on the left of the casualty with his palm upwards and holding a folded handkerchief to prevent hurting by the finger nails, the First Aider on the right of the casualty with his palms downwards, (hook-grip).

The First Aiders rise together and step off with outside feet.

In all cases of carrying by hand seats the cross-over step and not side paces will be used.

Kitchen chair method

When a casualty, conscious and without serious injuries, is to be moved up or down stairs or along passageways, an ordinary kitchen-type chair can be used. The way should first of all be cleared of furniture or other obstruction.

The casualty should be seated on the chair and supported by

First Aiders, front and rear. The chair and the casualty are then slowly tilted backwards to an angle of 30° with the horizontal and lifted.

One First Aider should support the back of the chair and the casualty; the other, facing the casualty, should hold the chair by the front legs and move carefully backwards down the stairs.

If the stairs or passageway are wide enough, the First Aiders can stand at the sides of the chair, each supporting a back and front leg of the chair.

Blanket lift

This method is described on page 117

Stretchers

Stretchers in common use are of two patterns, viz: 'Ordinary' and 'Telescopic-handled'.

In principle they are alike, the component parts being designated the poles, handles, traverses, runners and canvas bed. The 'head' and 'foot' of a stretcher correspond to the head and feet of the casualty.

At the head of the bed there may be a canvas overlay (the pillow-sack) which can be filled with soft material to form a pillow. It opens at the head and its contents can be adjusted without unduly disturbing the casualty.

The traverses are provided with joints for opening and closing the stretcher.

The length of the telescopic-handled pattern can be reduced to 6 feet by sliding the handles beneath the poles. This is of great value when working in confined areas.

When closed, the poles lie close together with the traverses being bent inwards. The canvas bed is folded on top of the poles and held in position by two transverse straps. If slings are carried they are laid along the canvas and secured by the straps round the poles and bed.

Preparing and blanketing a stretcher

On the command *'Prepare and blanket stretcher'* –
–two First Aiders will open and secure the stretcher, ensuring that the traverses are fully opened;
–the stretcher is then tested by one person lying on it and the

184

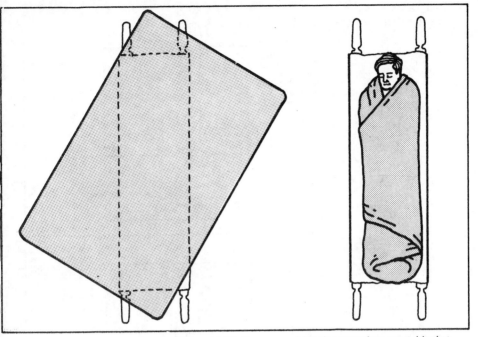

Figures 152 and 153: Prepare and blanket stretcher — one blanket

two ends of the stretcher raised off the ground in turn, to ensure the bed will take the weight of the casualty. Then the stretcher is blanketed according to the number of blankets available.

With one blanket   Place the blanket diagonally over the stretcher.

After placing the casualty on the stretcher —
—carry the point of the blanket at the head round his neck and on to his chest;
—the point of the blanket at the foot is brought up over the casualty's feet and a small fold tucked between the ankles to prevent rubbing;
—the right side of the blanket is carried over the casualty and tucked in;
—the left side of the blanket is brought over and tucked in.

With two blankets   Place the first blanket lengthwise across the stretcher with one edge covering half the handles at the head, and slightly more to one side of the stretcher than the other.

185

Figures 154, 155 and 156:
Prepare and blanket stretcher
– two blankets

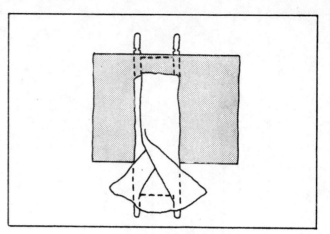

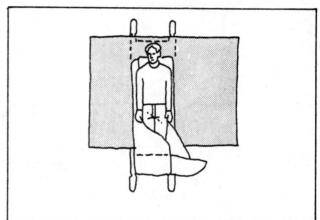

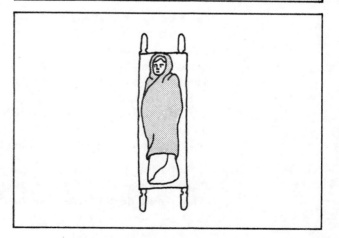

Figure 157: Blanket
lift: Preparation

Figure 158: Blanket lift:
Rolling on

Figure 159: Blanket lift:
Lifting

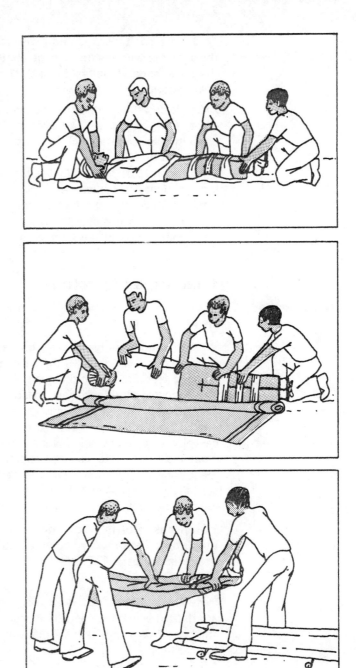

Fold the second blanket lengthwise into three and place on the stretcher with the upper edge about fifteen inches below the upper edge of the first blanket. Open out the folds at the lower end for about two feet.

After placing the casualty on the stretcher –
– the foot of the second blanket is brought over the casualty's feet and a small fold tucked between the ankles to prevent rubbing;
– the open folds of the blanket are then brought over the legs and feet and tucked in;
– the upper corners of the first blanket are turned in and the shorter side brought over the casualty and tucked in;
– the longer side of the blanket is then brought over and tucked in.

Loading a stretcher

Four bearers
A squad of four, numbered 1 to 4 are required. All orders are given by No. 1.

When casualty is lying on a blanket: The bearers place themselves on each side of the casualty, Nos. 1 and 2 at the feet and Nos. 3 and 4 at the head.
The edges of the blanket are rolled against the side of the casualty and each bearer firmly grasps the rolled edges with hands about six inches apart. At the command of No. 1, the casualty is carefully and evenly lifted and unless a fifth person is available to slide the stretcher under the casualty, the four bearers will move with short even side steps until the casualty is directly over the canvas bed. He is then gently lowered on to it.

When casualty is not lying on a blanket but one is available: The casualty should be placed on the blanket as described on page 117 and then lifted on to the stretcher as described above.

When casualty is not lying on a blanket and none is available: When the casualty is ready for loading on to the stretcher, Nos. 2, 3 and 4 will place themselves on the left of the casualty –
No. 2 facing the knees,
No. 3 facing the hips, and

gure 160: Loading
ithout a blanket:
osition of bearers

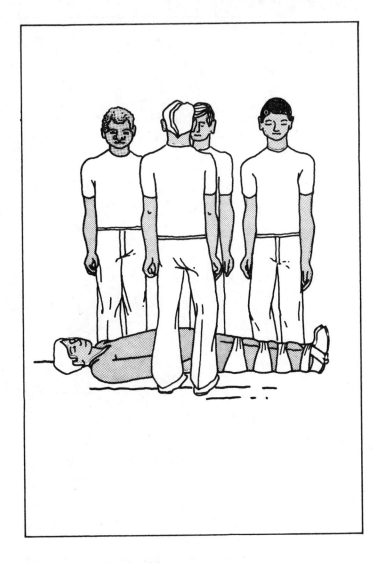

No. 4 facing the shoulders.

No. 1 will place himself on the right of the casualty facing No. 3.

All will go down on their left knees and place their forearms beneath the casualty paying particular attention to the site of the injury. Using the hook-grip, No. 1 joins his left hand with the left hand of No. 4 and his right hand with the right

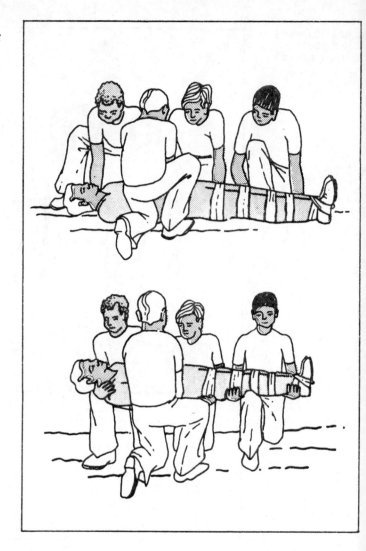

hand of No. 3. No. 4 supports the head and shoulders, No. 2 the lower limbs.

When No. 1 gives the order *'Lift'*, the casualty must be lifted gently, slowly and evenly and placed on the knees of Nos. 2, 3 and 4. No. 1 will disengage, get the prepared stretcher and place it under the casualty, so that when he is lowered on to it, his head will just be clear of the traverse at the top

*Figure 162: Loading
without a blanket:
Third and fourth moves*

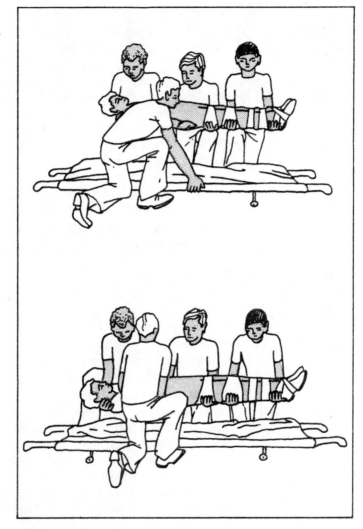

and will rest on the pillow. No. 1 will then resume his position
and rejoin hands with bearers Nos. 4 and 3.

When No. 1 gives the order *'Lower'*, the casualty will be
raised slightly from the knees of the bearers, and then
lowered gently, slowly and evenly on to the stretcher bed.
The bearers then rise and turn to face the foot of the stretcher.
If lifting the casualty from the right side, bearers go down on

their right knees.

Three bearers When only three bearers are available, the stretcher will be placed at the casualty's head in line with his body. No. 1 will kneel on the left knee on the injured side opposite the casualty's knees; he passes his hands under the casualty's legs; Nos. 2 and 3 kneel on their left knees on opposite sides of the casualty; they pass their hands under his shoulders and hips and lock their fingers in the hook-grip. On the command 'Lift', the bearers will rise to the erect position and, moving by side paces, carry the casualty head first over the foot of the stretcher, the horizontal position of his body being maintained throughout the movement. The casualty is then lowered carefully on the stretcher.

When unloading, the casualty will be uplifted and carried head foremost over the head of the stretcher.

Two bearers For use in mines and narrow cuttings where space is limited.

The stretcher will be placed at the casualty's head in line with his body. Both bearers will stand astride the casualty, No. 2 at the head, placing his forearms under the casualty's shoulders, No. 1 about the knees, placing his left hand beneath the casualty's thighs and his right below the knees. When both are ready No. 1 will give the command 'Lift'.

When the command 'Advance' is given both will step off together with the left foot, taking short even paces and stooping so that the body of the casualty is not far from the ground. They will advance until the casualty is over the stretcher, when No. 1 gives the order 'Halt–Lower'. The casualty is lowered gently on to the stretcher. Both bearers then take up position on the left of the stretcher ready for lifting, No. 2 at the head and No. 1 at the foot.

Carrying a stretcher

No. 1 will decide whether the stretcher is to be carried by four or two bearers. When the casualty has been placed on the stretcher, the bearers will take up their positions alongside the stretcher.

No. 1 at the foot of the stretcher on the right;
No. 2 at the foot of the stretcher on the left;

192

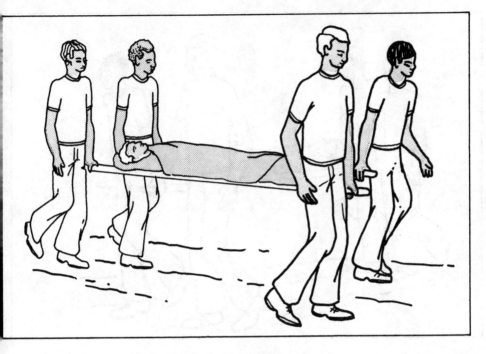

Figure 163: Hand carriage: Four bearers

No. 3 at the head of the stretcher on the right;
No. 4 at the head of the stretcher on the left.

By four bearers

On the command *'Hand carriage by four bearers'*, all four bearers will stoop together and grasp the handles with their inner hands. On the command *'Lift'*, the bearers will rise together, holding the stretcher at the full extent of their arms. At the command *'Advance'*, all bearers will step off with the inner foot, keeping their knees slightly bent and walking with a relaxed gait.

On the command *'Lower stretcher'*, the four bearers will stoop, gently lower the stretcher to the ground and then rise together.

By two bearers

On the command *'Hand carriage by two bearers'*, Nos. 2 and 4 will take side paces over the handles of the stretcher, and if slings are to be used, they will place them over their shoulders and on the handles of the stretcher. On the

193

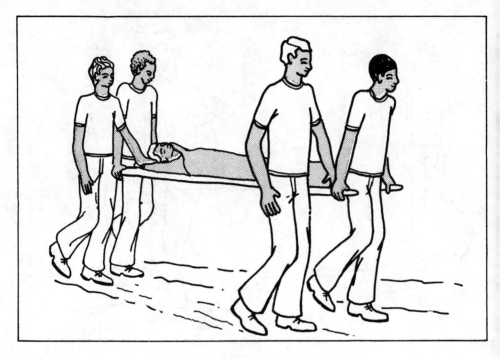

Figure 164: Hand carriage: Two bearers

command *'Lift'*, the two bearers will rise together keeping the stretcher level. Nos. 1 and 3 will turn inwards to assist. No. 1 particularly can help to prevent the casualty's feet catching the buttocks of No. 2.

On the command *'Adjust slings'*, Nos. 1 and 3 turn to the left and adjust the slings of Nos. 2 and 4 respectively.

On the command *'Advance'*, Nos. 1, 2 and 3 will step off with their left foot and No. 4 with his right. Bearers must keep their knees slightly bent and walk with a relaxed gait.

On the command *'Lower stretcher'*, Nos. 2 and 4 stoop slowly, evenly and gently lower the stretcher to the ground, then rise together. If slings are used Nos. 2 and 4 will remove them and after lowering the stretcher will step over the handles and take up their former positions, placing the loops of the folded slings over the near handles and the ends over the other handles.

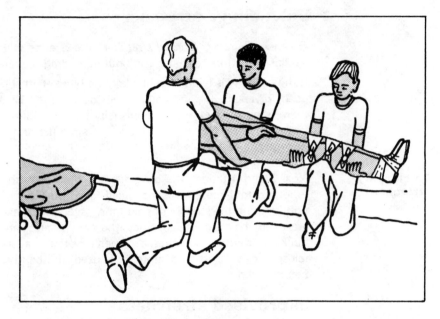

Figure 165: Three-bearer lift

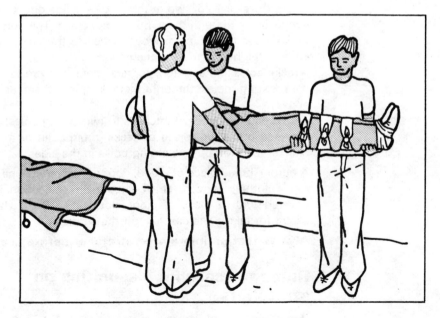

Figure 166: Three-bearer lift

195

Unloading a stretcher

On the command *'Unload stretcher'*, the bearers will adopt similar procedure to that carried out in loading the stretcher.

If the casualty is lying on a blanket, the blanket lift should be used, reversing the method described on page 117. Where there is no blanket, after the casualty has been lifted to the bearers' knees, No. 1 will remove the stretcher and place it beyond the casualty's feet.

To close a stretcher

Nos. 2 and 4 unlock the traverses and then push the poles together, fold the canvas on itself and buckle the straps tightly round the stretcher behind the traverses. Where slings are used they are placed along the canvas and the straps buckled round the stretcher behind the traverses. If telescopic-handled type stretcher is used, the handles must be pushed home.

Improvised stretchers

Stretchers may be improvised as follows —
— turn the sleeves of two or three coats inside out; pass two strong poles through them, button the coats. The poles may be kept apart by strips of wood lashed to the poles at both ends of the bed formed by the coats;
— make holes in the bottom corners of one or more sacks and pass strong poles through them keeping them apart as above;
— tie broad bandages at intervals to two strong poles;
— spread out a rug, piece of sacking, tarpaulin or a strong blanket, and roll up two strong poles in the sides.

A hurdle, broad piece of wood, door or shutter may be used; rugs, clothing, hay or straw should be placed on it and covered with a piece of stout cloth or sacking which is useful for taking the casualty off the stretcher.

Always test an improvised stretcher before use.

Rules for carrying casualties on stretchers

As a general rule, the casualty is carried feet first. The

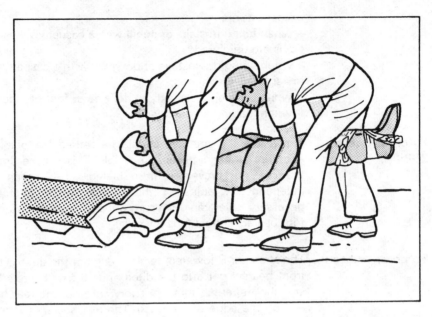

Figure 167: Two-bearer lift

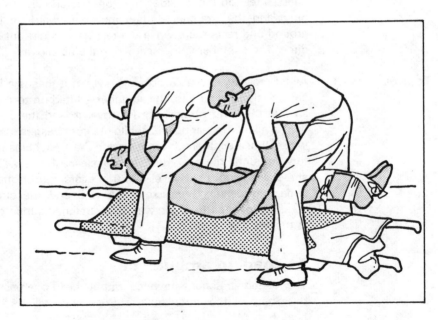

Figure 168: Two-bearer lift

exceptions are —
– when going upstairs or uphill with a casualty whose lower limbs are uninjured;
– when going downstairs or downhill with a casualty whose lower limbs are injured;
– when carrying a casualty to the side or foot of a bed;
– when loading an ambulance.

To cross uneven ground
If possible the stretcher should be carried by four bearers and kept as nearly level as possible. This can be done and the casualty prevented from falling off by each bearer independently adjusting the height of the stretcher as necessary. Over very uneven ground for a short distance the four bearers should face inwards.

To cross a ditch
The stretcher is lowered near the edge of the ditch. The two front bearers get into the ditch and all four bearers lift the stretcher together, moving it forward until the rear handles rest on the edge of the ditch. The rear bearers get into the ditch and the stretcher is then moved so that the front handles rest on the far side. The front bearers get out of the ditch and the stretcher is then moved forward on to the ground and rests there while the rear bearers get out of the ditch. The stretcher is then carried in the usual way.

To cross a wall
Avoid crossing a wall, if possible, even if it means a longer carry. If there is no gap, the stretcher is lifted on to the wall so that the front runners are just over it, and the stretcher held level by the rear bearers while the front bearers cross the wall. All bearers then lift together and the stretcher is moved forward until the rear runners are clear of the wall, the stretcher being held level by the bearers in front. The remaining bearers then cross the wall and the stretcher carefully lowered from the wall. The stretcher is then carried in the usual way.

To load an ambulance

The loaded stretcher is lowered with its head one pace from the doors of the ambulance. The casualty will be loaded head first.

The bearers now stand to the stretcher, Nos. 3 and 4 at the head, and Nos. 1 and 2 at the foot.

On the command 'Load', the bearers turn inwards, stoop, grasp the poles of the stretcher, hands wide apart, palms uppermost; they rise slowly, lifting the stretcher, holding it level at the full extent of the arms. They then take a side-pace to the ambulance, raising the stretcher evenly to the level of the compartment to be loaded. The front bearers place the runners in the grooves and then assist the rear bearers to slide the stretcher into its place and secure it. If slings have been used they should be kept with their stretcher.

Many ambulances are provided with upper and lower berths. In such cases the sequence of loading is upper right, upper left, lower right, lower left.

If the ambulance to be loaded is of the single rear door type, it should be loaded in the following manner. On the command 'Load', No. 4 will take up position inside the ambulance facing the stretcher and No. 2 will take up position opposite No. 3, with No. 1 between the handles facing the ambulance. Nos. 2 and 3 turn inwards and all three bearers lift the stretcher to the required height, move forward and hand the head of the stretcher to No. 4, Nos. 2 and 3 moving backwards to assist No. 1 who will load the appropriate berth with No. 4.

To unload an ambulance

Two bearers take hold of the handles at the rear and gently withdraw the stretcher. As it is withdrawn, the other two bearers will take hold of the handles at the front, and, taking the weight, lower it to the full extent of their arms, then by side paces march clear of the ambulance and lower the stretcher to the ground.

To unload an ambulance with a single door, Nos. 4 and 1 will enter the ambulance, with Nos. 2 and 3 on either side of the door to assist No. 1 to descend. The stretcher is then withdrawn from the ambulance, and Nos. 2 and 3 receive the head of the stretcher from No. 4. The stretcher is then carried clear of the ambulance and lowered to the ground.

199

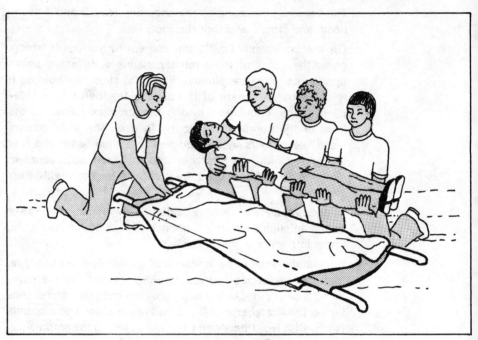

Figure 169: Transferring casualty from stretcher

Transferring the casualty from a stretcher on to a bed (or examination couch)

From the foot of the bed

The head of the stretcher is lifted so that the fore runners are in front of the rail at the foot of the bed (or well on to the couch).

The casualty is lifted by Nos. 2, 3 and 4 bearers. No. 1 bearer then removes the stretcher. By short paces to the side, Nos' 2, 3 and 4 bearers carry the casualty to the required place. He is then lowered and put in a suitable position.

The casualty's boots or shoes are removed;
– the covering or bedding is adjusted;
– the casualty is given a urine bottle if required.

From the floor

The stretcher is lowered at the side of the bed or couch.

Nos. 2, 3 and 4 bearers will take positions on the side farthest from the bed or couch, No. 1 being opposite No. 3.

The casualty is lifted from the stretcher on the right or left knees of the three bearers, while No. 1 disengages and removes the stretcher. He then joins hands with No. 3 and all bearers rise to a standing position, supporting the casualty on their forearms. No. 1 disengages and goes to the casualty's head and supports it.

All bearers then step forward and gently place the casualty on the bed or couch.

Emergency Resuscitation

Silvester method

If ventilation of the lungs by the expired air method cannot be undertaken because of facial injuries or for some other reason, the Silvester method is recommended as an alternative, as it allows external cardiac compression to be used also when necessary.

Treatment

1. Remove any obvious obstruction from the mouth.

2. Lay the casualty on his back on a firm surface.

3. Raise his shoulders on a folded jacket or in some other way.

4. Check that the airway is clear by extending the head backwards.

5. Kneel astride the casualty's head.

6. If necessary, turn his head to one side to clear out the mouth.

7. Grasp his wrists, cross them over the lower part of his chest.

8. Rock your body forward and press down on the casualty's chest (Figure 170).

9. Release the pressure and with a sweeping movement, draw the casualty's arms backwards and outwards as far as possible (Figures 171 and 172).

10. Repeat the procedure rhythmically (twelve times per minute in the adult).

If no improvement is noticed in the colour and appearance of the casualty, turn him on his side and strike him smartly on the back between the shoulders to clear any obstruction. Re-commence the cycle.

Figures 170, 171 and 172:
Silvester method of
emergency resuscitation

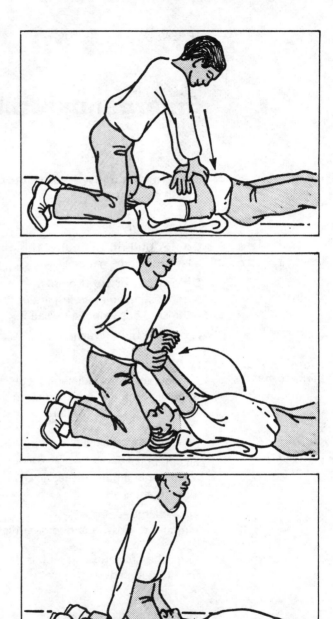

203

Emergency Childbirth

General rules

Send for the midwife or doctor; meantime –
– keep calm;
– let nature take its course;
– do not hurry.

Do not pull on the baby, the cord, or the afterbirth –
– let them come naturally.

Do not cut or tie the cord –
– until baby and afterbirth are *both* delivered *or*
– the cord has stopped pulsating.

Keep the baby warm.

Signs and symptoms

Low backache.
A 'show' of blood-stained mucus.
Regular contractions occurring in the lower abdomen.
The 'breaking of the waters' (occasionally).

Outline of treatment

Reassure the prospective mother.

Ensure privacy –
– put her in a quiet place;
– keep others away.

Take charge –
– until the midwife or doctor arrives.

Preparation

From the first sign that labour has started there is plenty of time to get ready.

Don't fuss.

Get a cot ready for the baby –
– a basket, box or drawer.

He will need a blanket, shawl or towel to keep him warm.
Keep him out of draughts and the cold.

Have ready scissors (boiled for 10 minutes) to cut the cord.

If no sterile ligatures are available boil (10 minutes), or soak in methylated spirit (10 minutes), three pieces of string nine inches long –
– these are for tying the cord.

If no bed is available prepare a clean surface for the mother to lie on –
– protect the bed or surface with a sheet of plastic material or newspapers and cover with a clean towel or sheet.

Take a blanket, fold into three, top to bottom, wrap it in a clean sheet – this makes a pack to cover the top half of the mother's body.

Have jugs of hot water available and clean basins, also a plastic or stout paper bag to hold soiled swabs, etc.

Prevention of infection

Infection or dirt is a grave danger to mother and baby.

No person who has a cold, sore throat, or septic hands, should help.

Lack of scrupulous cleanliness will jeopardise the life of mother and child.

You and your assistant should wear masks –
– improvise with a clean handkerchief.

Scrub your nails and wash your hands thoroughly, if possible under running water for four minutes.

Do not dry them.

If they get soiled, wash again.

First stage

The uterus contracts every 10 to 20 minutes –
– Normally the stage may last for several hours.
– the contractions are dilating the neck of the uterus and the birth canal.

Signs and symptoms

The 'show' of blood-stained mucus increases.

The cramp-like pains increase and last up to a minute –
– as the birth progresses they become more frequent.

Second stage

May start with the 'breaking of the waters' surrounding the baby.

205

A pint or more of water gushes out –
– this means that the baby is on its way.

During the early part of this stage the mother may be kept on her back.

During the contractions she should draw her knees up, holding them with her hands, bend her head forward and hold her breath. She should rest as much as possible between contractions.

Treatment

When a bulge appears –

1. Turn the mother on to her left side.

2. Instruct her to draw her knees up, with her buttocks near to the edge of the bed.

3. Keep her body warm.

4. Support her head with a pillow.

Should a bowel movement occur **beware of soiling the birth canal.**

Wipe clean from in front backwards.

The birth

The mother should **not bear down during the contractions; nor hold her breath.**

She should keep her mouth open and pant, i.e., take short breaths, so that the baby may emerge **slowly.**

The head commonly emerges first with the face looking back. The bottom, foot or arm may appear first.

Do not interfere unless –
– a membrane is over the face – it must be torn;
– the cord is around the baby's neck – try to ease it over the head or loop it over the shoulder.

Do not pull the baby or the cord – if the cord is pulled and the placenta is torn the baby may bleed to death.

Support the baby's head in the palms of your hands and wait.

The next contraction delivers the baby's shoulders.

Get hold of its body under the armpits and lift the baby towards its mother's abdomen.

Lay the baby by the mother's legs with the head lower than the body.

Ensure that the cord is not stretched.

Immediate care of the baby

Remember he is wet and very slippery.

1. Wrap a cloth round his ankles.

2. Take a good grip with one finger between the ankles.

3. Hold him up head downwards.

4. Allow any fluid to drain from his mouth and nose by holding with his head slightly back and opening his mouth.

5. With a clean piece of cloth or gauze gently wipe away any blood or mucus from the baby's mouth and throat.

6. When the baby cries lay him on his side close to his mother, not face downwards.

Should he not cry nor show signs of breathing *in two minutes,* **start resuscitation,** by ventilating his lungs, blowing *very gently.*

On no account should the baby be handled roughly or smacked.

Breech delivery

Should the baby appear bottom first, *no interference* is the rule.

Only after the shoulders have emerged and the head retained for three minutes may gentle traction be necessary.

Third stage

The afterbirth will be expelled by uterine contractions and the mother's voluntary efforts.

So turn the mother on her back and separate her legs.

Ten or more minutes may elapse before the afterbirth appears.

If there is much bleeding gently massage the top of the uterus which is found just below the navel – it will stimulate it to contract.

Keep the Afterbirth – it is required for checking that it is complete.

207

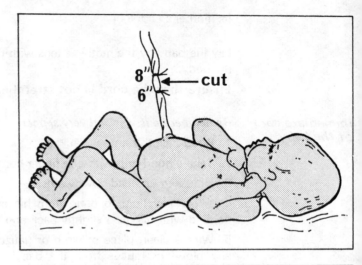

Figure 173: The umbilical cord: position of first and second knots

8"
6"
← cut

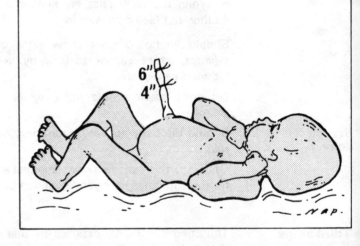

Figure 174: The umbilical cord: position of third knot

6"
4"

Dealing with the cord

Wait until –
– the afterbirth has been delivered *or*
– the cord has stopped pulsating, *or*
– ten minutes have elapsed since the birth of the baby.

Tie the cord very firmly in two places –
– one six inches and one eight inches from the baby's navel.

Unless the cord on the baby's side is securely tied he may bleed to death.

208

Cut the cord between the two ties (Figure 173).

No powder or disinfectant of any kind should be put on the cord or navel.

Place a sterile dressing over the cut end at the baby's navel.

Inspect the baby's cord ten minutes after cutting to see that there is no bleeding. Tie the cord again securely four inches from the baby's navel (Figure 174).

Re-dress the cord and secure by wrapping a binder or folded napkin around the baby.

If a sterile dressing is not available, no dressing or binder should be used.

If the afterbirth has not yet been expelled, cover the end of the umbilical cord attached to it with a sterile dressing and tie it in place.

Care of the mother

Wash the mother and fix a sanitary towel in position.

Give her hot drinks, biscuits, etc.

Encourage her to sleep.

Check her pulse and respiration rates.

First Aid equipment in the home

An adequate supply of dressings should be available in the home. The minimum required under the terms of the Offices, Shops and Railway Premises Order 1964 (Statutory Instrument 1964 No. 970), in the United Kingdom, where the number of people does not exceed ten, may be taken as a guide.

Sterilised unmedicated dressings –
– small;
– medium;
– large.

Adhesive wound dressings (assorted sizes) .. 12

Triangular bandage of unbleached calico, the longest side of which measures not less than 51 inches and each of the other sides not less than 36 inches .. 1

Adhesive plaster – 1 in × 5 yards .. .. .. 1 spool

½-oz packet of absorbent sterilised cotton wool .. 1

Sterilised eye-pad with bandage in sealed packet 1

Safety pins (assorted sizes) 6

In offices and industry

In the United Kingdom, this is covered by various Orders and Regulations issued by the Ministry of Labour, and employers are advised to obtain the relevant Order governing their premises. Similar legislation exists in other countries.

List of illustrations

211

212

214

Index

215

INDEX

INDEX

INDEX

INDEX

PULSE

Adult	60/80 (average 72)
Children	90/104

TEMPERATURES

Adult	97. 2 to 99. 5f

RATE OF BREATHING

Adult	15/18 per minute
Children	24/40 per minute
Liver	Right Side Upper part of abdomen by lower ribs
Spleen	Covered by Ribs upper part left side
Pancreas	Behind Stomach
Kidneys	At back region of Loins
Bladder	Front of Pelvis